AF734549

ENDOCRINOLOGY RESEARCH AND CLINICAL DEVELOPMENTS

ETHNICITY AND SYNDROME X

ENDOCRINOLOGY RESEARCH AND CLINICAL DEVELOPMENTS

Additional books and e-books in this series can be found on Nova's website under the Series tab.

ENDOCRINOLOGY RESEARCH AND CLINICAL DEVELOPMENTS

ETHNICITY AND SYNDROME X

MITHUN DAS, PHD
AND
KAUSHIK BOSE, PHD, DSC
EDITORS

nova
Medicine & Health
New York

Copyright © 2020 by Nova Science Publishers, Inc.

All rights reserved. No part of this book may be reproduced, stored in a retrieval system or transmitted in any form or by any means: electronic, electrostatic, magnetic, tape, mechanical photocopying, recording or otherwise without the written permission of the Publisher.

We have partnered with Copyright Clearance Center to make it easy for you to obtain permissions to reuse content from this publication. Simply navigate to this publication's page on Nova's website and locate the "Get Permission" button below the title description. This button is linked directly to the title's permission page on copyright.com. Alternatively, you can visit copyright.com and search by title, ISBN, or ISSN.

For further questions about using the service on copyright.com, please contact:
Copyright Clearance Center
Phone: +1-(978) 750-8400 Fax: +1-(978) 750-4470 E-mail: info@copyright.com.

NOTICE TO THE READER

The Publisher has taken reasonable care in the preparation of this book, but makes no expressed or implied warranty of any kind and assumes no responsibility for any errors or omissions. No liability is assumed for incidental or consequential damages in connection with or arising out of information contained in this book. The Publisher shall not be liable for any special, consequential, or exemplary damages resulting, in whole or in part, from the readers' use of, or reliance upon, this material. Any parts of this book based on government reports are so indicated and copyright is claimed for those parts to the extent applicable to compilations of such works.

Independent verification should be sought for any data, advice or recommendations contained in this book. In addition, no responsibility is assumed by the Publisher for any injury and/or damage to persons or property arising from any methods, products, instructions, ideas or otherwise contained in this publication.

This publication is designed to provide accurate and authoritative information with regard to the subject matter covered herein. It is sold with the clear understanding that the Publisher is not engaged in rendering legal or any other professional services. If legal or any other expert assistance is required, the services of a competent person should be sought. FROM A DECLARATION OF PARTICIPANTS JOINTLY ADOPTED BY A COMMITTEE OF THE AMERICAN BAR ASSOCIATION AND A COMMITTEE OF PUBLISHERS.

Additional color graphics may be available in the e-book version of this book.

Library of Congress Cataloging-in-Publication Data

ISBN: 978-1-53618-042-8
Library of Congress Control Number: 2020938365

Published by Nova Science Publishers, Inc. † New York

CONTENTS

Foreword **ix**
Sławomir Kozieł

Preface **xi**

Chapter 1 Ethnicity and Syndrome X **1**
Mithun Das and Kaushik Bose

Chapter 2 Transnational Migration as a Risk Factor for Syndrome X **25**
Sylvia Kirchengast

Chapter 3 Ethnic Diversities and Risk Factors with Syndrome X in South Africa **47**
Yackoob Kassim Seedat

Chapter 4 A Comparative Study on Nutritional Status among Tribal and Non-Tribal Mothers in Rajshahi District Bangladesh: A Cross-Sectional Study **57**
Md. Masud Rana, Md. Reazul Karim, Md. Rafiqul Islam, Premananda Bharati and Md. Golam Hossain

Chapter 5	Comparative Analysis of Total Body Parameters and Functional Characteristics of Mongolian Rural and Urban Children and Adolescents *Elena Z. Godina, L. Gundegmaa and Ekaterina Yu. Permiakova*	**75**
Chapter 6	Metabolic Syndrome among Indian Females: A Review *Ramanpreet Randhawa and Sharda Sidhu*	**93**
Chapter 7	Prevalence of Undernutrition, Obesity and Hypertension among Adult Shabars and Mahalis of Bankura District of West Bengal, India *Shilpita Bhandari, Sadaruddin Biswas, Mihir Ghosh, Binoy Kumar Kuiti and Kaushik Bose*	**113**
Chapter 8	Effect of Human Migration on Hypertension, Cardiovascular Diseases, Type 2 Diabetes and Their Associations with Metabolic Syndrome among the Asian Indians *Nitish Mondal and Jaydip Sen*	**129**
Chapter 9	Ethnic Differences in Proinflammatory State and Syndrome X: An Overview *Plaban Chaudhury, Riddhi Goswami and Mithun Das*	**153**
Chapter 10	Anthropometric Measures, Body Composition and the Risk of Hypertension: A Study on Indian Tribes *Gautam Kumar Kshatriya and Anjali Kumari*	**163**
Chapter 11	Cardio-Metabolic Risk among the High Altitude Inhabitants: A Brief Review *Sovanjan Sarkar and Mithun Das*	**181**

Editors' Contact Information 199

Index 201

FOREWORD

Despite the growing efforts of preventive medicine and public health obesity still remains as a major problem and the number of obese people is increasing. However, the main objective in strife of obesity should not be obesity *per se* but rather its metabolic consequences called syndrome X. This syndrome to be often called a silent killer, which after 5-15 years, giving no symptoms in seemingly healthy people, leads to development of diabetes, atherosclerosis, heart attack and stroke. But the list of health complications after syndrome X is much longer, and among them it should be mentioned osteoporosis, initial fatty liver, night apnoea syndrome, depression, in females too high androgens level and intensification free radical production. Some authors have pointed out that high level of insulin, as a corollary of metabolic disorders, increases a risk of colon malignant tumours.

First noticed that civilization diseases can begin metabolic disorders appeared more than 90 years ago, but in 1988 year Prof. Gerald Reaven from Stanford University used as a first a term "syndrome X", and in 1998 year metabolic disorders were registered as a disease entity by World Health Organisation.

The main symptom of metabolic syndrome is an abdominal obesity and two from four accompanying factors like increased level of triglycerides and glucose, lower level of HDL cholesterol fraction and hypertension. The cause of syndrome X are definitely excessive food consumption and physical inactivity, however some research indicated that metabolic disorders occur in ever fourth person with only insignificant overweight. Especially persons born with low birth weight and/or overfed during infancy and early childhood are prone to suffer from metabolic disorders in adulthood. Genetic predisposition plays an important role. It is assumed that 250 genes are responsible for development of obesity and syndrome X.

In the day of globalisation related to spreading the western style of life and eating behaviour makes various ethnic groups particularly vulnerable. Preserved for dozens of generations traditional life style and nutritional behaviour very often is destroyed facing a meeting with western civilisation. This departure from tradition leads inevitably to health consequences.

The edited book entitled "Ethnicity and Syndrome X" is an excellent review of this issue and consists of eleven research manuscripts bringing the reader closer to ethnic diversities in relation to syndrome X in South Africa, Bangladesh, Mongolia, India, and among Asian Indians including high altitude inhabitants all over the World. This knowledge compendium indicates important significance of conductive factors of development of syndrome X like transnational migration (chapter 2), ethnic diversity (chapter 3), nutritional status (Chapter 4), body parameters and functional characteristics (chapter 5), sex (chapter 6), prevalence of burden of diseases and hypertension (chapter 7), human migration and hypertension (chapter 8), effect of C-reactive protein and family history (chapter 9), body composition and body parameters and the risk of hypertension (chapter 10), and reports worldwide prevalence of metabolic syndrome among high altitude inhabitants (Chapter 11).

All manuscripts were contributed by eminent anthropologist, tribal researchers and genetics. It makes this volume extremely stimulative and useful providing wide-ranging directions for further studies.

Prof. Sławomir Kozieł
Department of Anthropology,
Hirszfeld Institute of Immunology and Experimental Therapy,
Polish Academy of Sciences,
Wroclaw, Poland
e-mail: slawomir.koziel@hirszfeld.pl

PREFACE

The syndrome X or metabolic syndrome may be defined as a constellation of several interrelated risk factors of metabolic origin which includes centrally distributed obesity, decreased high density lipoprotein cholesterol, elevated triglycerides, elevated blood pressure and hyperglycemia. Persons with syndrome X are at twice the risk of developing cardiovascular disease, and are at about five-fold the risk of type 2 diabetes mellitus as compare to persons with this syndrome.

There are considerable evidences of important ethnic differences in the prevalence of syndrome X, its components and sequelae. The prevalence varied between ethnic groups even within the same geographical location. Apart from multifactorial (genetic vs. environmental) nature, there are intriguing metabolic and anthropometric differences found across different ethnic groups. The estimates vary by ethnicity, for instance, high prevalence in non-European groups such as Black African-Caribbeans, Hispanics, indigenous populations of North America, South Asians, and the Western Pacific Region and lower prevalence in Chinese populations, and European-White.

Public health strategies that are well known to be important for chronic disease prevention in general can substantially reduce the prevalence of syndrome X. Population-specific studies will be important in identifying subgroups for which syndrome X is a health issue and for which disease management strategies are needed. Simultaneously, studies to identify different biomarkers associated with syndrome X that are linked with the development of specific chronic diseases, such as CVD and diabetes, will significantly enhance the early detection of these diseases. Existing preventions strategies, if implemented in population subgroups at highest risk, may have a substantial effect on reducing these trends. The prevalence of syndrome X increases with advancing age suggests that the efforts to increase awareness of prevention strategies must begin early. Intensive treatment and effective targeting efforts would help in avoiding future sequelae of syndrome X across different ethnicity.

This book will be an assemblage of similarities and differences in the risk of syndrome X and related disorders among different ethnic groups worldwide, and reviews potential mechanisms for ethnic differences. It would certain help in translational research for early intervention and better prevention of syndrome X and its associated public health burden worldwide.

Dr. Mithun Das, Ph.D. (Visva-Bharati)
Prof. Kaushik Bose, Ph.D. (Punjab), Ph.D. (Cantab), D.Sc. (Vidyasagar)

In: Ethnicity and Syndrome X
Editors: M. Das and K. Bose
ISBN: 978-1-53618-042-8
© 2020 Nova Science Publishers, Inc.

Chapter 1

ETHNICITY AND SYNDROME X

Mithun Das[1,*] and Kaushik Bose[2]
[1]Department of Anthropology, Sidho-Kanho-Birsha University, Purulia, West Bengal, India
[2]Department of Anthropology, Vidyasagar University, Midnapore, West Bengal, India

INTRODUCTION

The Syndrome X or metabolic syndrome may be defined as the constellation of interrelated risk factors of metabolic origin (Grundy, 2005). The constellation of centrally distributed obesity, decreased high density lipoprotein cholesterol (HDLc), elevated triglycerides, elevated blood pressures, and hyperglycemia is known as the Syndrome X (Zimmet et al., 2005). Person with this syndrome are at essentially twice the risk for cardiovascular disease (CVD) and further raises the risk for type 2 diabetes mellitus (T2DM) by about five-fold as compared with those without the syndrome (Grundy, 2007). In most countries, about 20-30% of the adult

*Corresponding Author's Email: mithundas01@yahoo.com.

population is predisposed to syndrome X (Grundy, 2008). It is not a discrete entity known to be caused by a single factor. Moreover, it shows considerable variation in the components among different individuals. This variation is even greater among different ethnic groups across the globe (Grundy et al., 2005). It is not restricted to the adults only, the predisposition, however, starts much early in life especially during the adolescent and young age. (Smith & Essop, 2009; Nelson & Bremer, 2010; Tailor et al., 2010).

The specific syndrome X components differ by ethnicity and gender. For instance, Hispanics were more likely to have high fasting glucose than the other ethnic groups. The presence of low HDLc was substantially lower among the black students than among the other two ethnic groups. Male adolescents were more likely to have low HDLc, high blood pressure, and high fasting glucose than female adolescents. These findings, collectively suggest that understanding the presence of the individual components of the syndrome by participant characteristics is important in order to make prevention efforts more successful across different ethnic and sex groups (STOPP-T2D, 2008). In Dallas Heart Study the variable manifestations of the components of the syndrome in white, black, and Hispanic men and women were studied (Victor et al., 2004). It showed that increasing waist girth is associated with a rise in all metabolic risk factors in black, white, and Hispanic men and women. The metabolic risk factors accompanying increased adipose tissue are believed to be related to abnormal production by adipose tissue of non-esterified fatty acids (NEFA) and other adipokines, such as adiponectin and inflammatory cytokines (Eckel et al., 2010). An important observation in this study was that among those with high waist girth, or what is called abdominal obesity in the United States, only about one-half or less had categorical metabolic risk factors. These findings however, do not minimize the impact of abdominal obesity on metabolic risk factors for the population as a whole, but they do show the importance of individual variability in susceptibility for their development.

Different threshold values have been set in different regions of the world. The threshold for abdominal obesity is set at a lower level, typically being 90–94 cm for men and 80 cm for women. Among South Asian, the cut-off for men is ≥ 90 cm and for women ≥ 80 cm. The overall intermediate waist girth is in the range of 90–101 cm for men and 80–90 cm for women. These ranges correspond closely to a body mass index (BMI) range of 25–29.9 kg/m^2. In this intermediate category, metabolic risk factors were more common than in those with low waist girths, but, on the whole, they were less prevalent than in subjects with high waist girths. These findings nonetheless add support for including intermediate waist girth in the definition of abdominal obesity, as advocated by some investigators. Yet such a definition must be made with an understanding that susceptibility for developing metabolic risk factors are indicative of high metabolic risk (Rosenzweig et al., 2008), or the syndrome X (Grundy et al., 2005). In a study, a high metabolic risk was relatively uncommon at intermediate waist girth except in Hispanic men. At high waist girth, three or more metabolic risk factors averaged about 30% in men and less than 20% in women. It raised the question of whether obesity should be considered more of a susceptibility factor for syndrome X than as a component of it (Vega et al., 2010). If not, obesity could be one of several factors, such as gender and ethnicity, as underlying susceptibility factors for the syndrome X.

First, variability in susceptibility to metabolic risk factors among waist girths, gender, and ethnicities is considerable although poorly understood. Whether these difference can be explained by genetic influences; environmental factors; or both remains to be elucidated. Second, there is a reasonable argument for including intermediate waist girth in the definition of abdominal obesity; on the other hand, metabolic risk factors are consistently higher in those with a high waist girth. Any definition of abdominal obesity thus depends on arbitrary considerations (Grundy et al., 2014). It was observed that the prevalence of the syndrome X was different, depending on the three definitions used. Moreover, the prevalence of elevated triglyceride levels (hypertriglyceridaemia), which is a distinctive feature of people of Indian origin, varied considerably in the study population owing to the use of the south Asian-specific (SAS) cut-off value for elevated triglycerides. The marked difference in the overall prevalence of the syndrome X from the ATP III (2005) definition to the SAS (2009) definition (48.3 vs31.4%) was due to the use of the south Asian-specific cut-off values for waist girth and triglyceride levels. Importantly, whether the modified ATP III (2005) or the revised SAS (2009) definition is used, a large number of individuals are likely to be misclassified due to lack of a common minimum criterion required to better comprehend the problem of the syndrome X among Asian Indians (Das et al., 2011). Several other studies have shown such discrepancies, not only in the Indian population but also in other Asian countries, such as China and Iran. In a study from India, the World Health Organisation (WHO), ATP III and IDF criteria of the syndrome X identified a differential prevalence of the syndrome in the population studied.The WHO criteria identified a greater number of coronary artery disease (CAD) subjects in males, but not in females (Deepa et al., 2007). Studies pertaining to Asian Indians revealed that the ATP III criteria identified a significantly higher proportion of people with the syndrome compared with the WHO criteria (Kanjilal et al., 2008; Wasir et al., 2008). It was mentioned that lower cut-off values of waist girth and BMI to define the MS might be critical for the accurate assessment of the MS among Asian Indians. Moreover, inclusion of BMI and making waist girth a non-obligatory criterion, more cases of the syndrome X were detected. However, for Asian Indians, making waist girth a mandatory variable to define the syndrome would lead to non-inclusion of many patients who would otherwise be diagnosed as having the syndrome according to the modified NCEP ATP III definition. A study from China also revealed that in subjects with established T2DM, the International Diabetes Federation (IDF) definition of the syndrome failed to identify a subgroup of patients who had the highest risk for coronary heart disease (CHD), whereas the ATP III definition predicted an increased risk of CHD in the same cohort (Tong et al., 2007). In a study in an adult Iranian population, the IDF definition of the syndrome was found to have a good correlation with the ATP III definition but a lower correlation with the WHO definition. It is therefore reasonable to argue that to use the presence of the syndrome X as a more sensitive guideline, factors such as family history of CVD, lack of physical activity, abuse of alcohol, cigarette smoking and tobacco chewing, along with region-specific cut-off values are required to better comprehend the syndrome X in people of Indian origin. There is an urgent need to develop a comprehensive risk profile for Asian Indians (Das et al., 2011).

Communicable Diseases to Non-Communicable Diseases: The Paradigm Shift

In developing countries, with improvement in economic situation there is an increasing prevalence of obesity and the syndrome X is seen in adults and more particularly in children. The main causes are increasing urbanization, change in dietary habits, and reduced physical activity. Furthermore, aggressive community nutrition intervention programs for undernourished children may increase obesity. Some evidence suggests that widely prevalent perinatal undernutrition and childhood catch-up obesity may play a role in adult-onset of syndrome X and T2DM. The economic cost of obesity and related diseases in developing countries, having meager health budgets is enormous (Misra & Khurana, 2008).

Modernization vis-à-vis Urbanization

Urbanization is the prime driver for nutrition transition and emergence of obesity, the syndrome X, and other non communicable diseases (NCDs) in developing countries. Remarkably, in 1999, when the world population was nearly 6 billion, a minimal increase in the populations of developed countries (1.9 to 1.21 billion) was seen compared with those of developing countries (4.87 to 6.9 billion), (Hoffman 2001), which were increasingly becoming urbanized. Urbanization is variable within developing regions: almost three fourths of the population in Latin America and the Caribbean, whereas 38% in Africa and Asia are urbanized (FAO 2004). The latter two regions are projected to have almost 50% urbanization by 2020. The rural-to-urban migration in many of the developing countries exposes migrants to urbanized diets and lifestyle. Studies done in Brazil and India have clearly shown that many of these migrants, now living in urban slums and city shanty towns, have become obese and also manifest a number of other cardiovascular risk factors (Misra & Khurana, 2008).

RAPID CHANGE IN DIETARY HABITS (THE NUTRITION TRANSITION)

Five patterns of nutrition transition, derived from historical references of human development, are present and evolve from one category to another in many ethnic groups and disparate geographical locations in developing countries. Pattern 1 nutrition transition is characteristic of hunter-gatherer populations and comprises diets rich in carbohydrates and fiber and low in fat, especially saturated fat, with a high-activity profile and lean body phenotype. In pattern 2, individuals exist in famine-like situation (low calorie, low protein and fat diets) and have growth retardation and low body fat and fat-free mass. In pattern 3, famine vanes, and nutrition improves, with increase in the consumption of fruits, vegetables, and animal proteins, and this pattern is associated with increasing inactivity. Pattern 4 is now most prevalent in developing countries, conducive to development of obesity, syndrome X, T2DM, and CVD. With improvement in economy, people become affluent and consume diets high in saturated fats, cholesterol, and refined carbohydrates and low in polyunsaturated fatty acids and fiber, associated with markedly sedentary lifestyle and increased stress. In the last (pattern 5), as people suffering from T2DM and CVD increase in the population, awareness of benefits of balanced diets and regular physical activity increases. Consequently, people attempt to change dietary and physical activity profiles to prevent or delay diseases. This pattern, unlike previous patterns, is driven by an individual's desire to seek healthy behavior, hence may not be evident in large segments of populations, and is likely to be adapted initially by affluent people. Furthermore, impetus to such lifestyle changes may be provided by government's policies, legal actions, and peer practices and hence may vary widely within each country. A rather rapid shift from pattern 3 to 4 in the developing countries is clearly responsible for steep increase in obesity and the syndrome X. As gross domestic product (GDP) of the country increases with improved economy, underweight children decrease, whereas overweight increases predominantly due to nutrition transition (Misra & Khurana, 2008).

Most developing countries in Asia, Latin America, Northern Africa, the Middle East, and the urban areas of sub-Saharan Africa have been experiencing a shift in the dietary patterns over the last few decades. Major dietary changes include a large increase in the consumption of fats, particularly animal fat and added sugar and decrease in cereal and fiber intake. Marked increase in the consumption of egg, poultry, pork, mutton, beef, and milk amounting to 1300 kcal/d has been reported in Chinese adults, proportional to increase in the income in China (Popkin & Du, 2003). In India and other South Asian countries, high intake of dairy products, sugar, and hydrogenated vegetable oils (e.g., vanaspati) is widely prevalent (Popkin, 2001). Availability of edible vegetable oils for consumption has nearly tripled throughout the developing world (FAO, 2004), For example, in China, availability of edible oils has risen 6-fold, whereas intake in the rest of Asia and Oceania tripled over the period from 1961 to 2000, much more than developed nations (FAO, 2004). Increased consumption of edible oils can be explained in part by rising demand but also import policies, as is evident in the three largest emerging economies, Brazil, China, and India (Hawkes, 2006). Importantly, consumption of nontraditional fast foods is occurring at a rapid pace in urban areas of several large cities in South Asia (Wasir & Misra, 2004). Locally made fast foods sold by street vendors in several developing countries, particularly in India and China, are equally unhealthy (Misra et al., 2008). These food items contain high amounts of trans-fatty acids due to deep frying in cheap and widely available hydrogenated vegetable oils.

Reduced Physical Activity

Occupational change, advent of newer technologies, and rapid pace of urban life have increasingly resulted in more sedentary work and less energy expenditure. Leisure time activities have also shifted from outdoor play to indoor entertainment; television viewing and computer games (Popkin, 2001). In the Philippines and China, shift to more passive commuting modes (i.e., increased motorized transportation) has increased physical inactivity

(Tudor-Locke et al., 2007). The household chores have become more mechanized with the use of multiple domestic automatic devices; microwave, improved food storage, washing machines, vacuum cleaners, etc., especially in India and China. Moreover, increasing mechanization even in rural areas (e.g., use of tractors than manual plowing of fields, use of motorized two-wheelers instead of bicycles) has contributed to physical inactivity in developing countries. Data from 212,021 adults from 51 countries, most of which were developing countries, in the World Health Survey (2002–2003) showed that about 15% of men and 20% of women were at risk for chronic diseases due to physical inactivity (Guthold et al., 2008). The prevalence of physical inactivity at less than the levels recommended for enhancing health was high in developing countries, ranging from 17 to91% (Oldridge, 2008). Remarkably, data from Brazil show that 70–80% of the populations are inactive (Matsudo et al., 2002). In Colombia, an estimated 7.6% of all-cause mortality and 20.1% of mortality due to chronic diseases were attributed to physical inactivity, and an estimated 5% of the mortality due to chronic diseases is preventable if physical inactivity was reduced by 30% (Lobelo et al., 2006). Physical inactivity contributed to 9.6% population-attributable risk and was an important risk factor for CVD in Costa Rica (Kabagambe et al., 2007). Finally, increase in obesity has been directly linked to physical inactivity in Chinese adults (Paeratakul et al., 1998; Popkin BM, 1999).

In most of the surveys, women are generally reported to be physically inactive than men, and this may also pertain to ethnic and cultural influences on outdoor activities. Physical inactivity was more prevalent in women than men in urban east India (85.4 *vs.* 75.4%) (Ghosh, 2006) and in Saudi Arabia (98.1 *vs.* 93.9%) (Al-Nozha et al., 2007). Immigrant women from the Middle East, including Iran and Turkey, had higher prevalence of abdominal obesity than Swedish- born women, with a high degree of physical inactivity during leisure time (Daryani et al., 2005). Of major concern is that children and adolescents are rapidly showing a decrease in physical activity levels, which is fueling obesity and T2DM at a young age. Urban Asian Indian adolescents who participated regularly in outdoor games had lower prevalence of overweight, with the risk being 3 times higher in those not participating in outdoor games (Laxmaiah, 2007). Only 22.4% of Saudi preschool children walked 10,000 steps or more per day (Al-Hazzaa & Al-Rasheedi, 2007). Nearly two thirds of Iranian adolescents aged 11–18 yr were physically inactive (Kelishadi et al., 2005). On account of cultural and weather barriers, adolescent girls had very low levels of physical activity in United Arab Emirates (Henry et al., 2004). Furthermore, non-obese Iranian children were reported to be more active in sports and went to school by foot compared with obese children who did not participate so much in sports and used mechanized transport (Mozaffari & Nabaei, 2007).

Growing Public Health Burden across the Globe

With a substantially high annual rate of increase of obesity and rapid emergence of the syndrome X in most developing countries, the shift in the pattern of NCDs is occurring at a faster rate than it did in the industrialized regions of the world half acentury ago (Popkin, 2002). Global prevalence of chronic diseases is projected to increase substantially over the next 2 decades in developing countries. Indeed, 60% of the global burden of chronic diseases is expected to occur in developing countries (Murray & Lopez, 1996). CVD is already the leading cause of mortality in many developing countries (WHO, 2008). In the World Health Report (1999), it was stated that in 1998, 78% of the burden of NCDs and 85% of the CVD arose from the developing low- and middle-income countries (WHO, 1999). Furthermore, according to projected data, chronic diseases will account for almost three quarters of all deaths worldwide by 2020 andthat 71% of deaths due to CVD and 70% of deaths due to diabetes will occur in developing countries (WHO, 1998). In fact, there are more patients with CVD in India and China than in all the economically developed countries (WHO, 2002). Globally, by 2000, 171 million patients with diabetes are projected, which is expected to increase to 366 million in 2030, of which 298 million will be in developing countries (15). The number of people with diabetes is projected to double (during 2000–2030), in three of the six developing regions, including, the Middle East and North Africa, South Asia, and sub-Saharan Africa (Wild et al., 2004). India has and will continue to have the highest number of patients with diabetes in the world (Sicree et al., 2006).

TRANSITION IN DEVELOPING COUNTRIES

Emergence of obesity and the syndrome X in developing countries is due to a number of factors; the most important are discussed below. Demographic transition (shift to low fertility, low mortality, and higher life expectancy) and epidemiologic transition (from widely prevalent infectious diseases to a pattern of high prevalence of chronic lifestyle related NCDs) have occurred in developing countries as they become economically more resourceful, socioeconomic transition (shift of people from low SES to high SES), causing significant shifts in dietary and physical activity patterns resulting in to nutrition and lifestyle transitions, and stress. These changes cause significant effects on body composition and metabolism, often resulting in increase in BMI, excess generalized and abdominal adiposity, deposition of ectopic fat, and increase in dyslipidemia and diabetes. Each type of transition has an important bearing on occurrence of obesity and metabolic risk factors; however, urbanization, nutrition transition, and increasing affluence remain the most important determinants of such dysmetabolic phenotype (Misra & Khurana, 2008).

THRIFTY GENOTYPE/THRIFTY PHENOTYPE HYPOTHESES

It is postulated that *thrifty* genotype is propagated by survival during famines and lends heightened tendency to develop obesity and T2DM seen in certain ethnic groups in developing countries with abundant food availability. This concept, although interesting, remains hypothetical and lacks firm evidence in the absence of definite identification of such thrifty genes (Prentice et al., 2005). Furthermore, natural selection by famine and tendency of individuals to gain weight with availability of abundant food should apply to the entire human population and should not be restricted to some sub-populations of developing countries (Prentice et al., 2005; Prentice, 2005). Moreover, different prevalence in obesity rates between genders and even between rural and urban-based populations belonging to low socio economic status (SES) indicate significant role of environmental and behavioral factors. Interestingly, in rural Gambia, children born low birth weight remained lean and largely free of metabolic diseases when they grew up as adults if they stayed in a rural setting and followed a frugal and traditional lifestyle (Moore et al., 2001; Prentice & Moore, 2005). These data show relative roles of genetic and environmental/ behavioral factors, suggesting that behavioral choices appear to be key mediators of development of obesity (Prentice, 2006).

A *thrifty* phenotype hypothesis that emphasizes fetal undernutrition leading to altered metabolic programing is perhaps a better explanation in resource-poor developing countries because abundant food supply later in life leads to maladaptive increase in weight and increases the risk of NCDs (Prentice & Moore, 2005; Prentice 2003; Hales & Barker, 2001). The evidence is available from many developing countries. Asian Indian babies born small and with low birth weight had higher systolic blood pressure and adiposity at 8 yr of age (Bavdekar et al., 1999). Chinese infants with low birth weight showed several cardiovascular risk factors at age 41–47 yr; hypertension, hyperglycemia, hyperinsulinemia, hypertriglyceridemia, and low levels of HDL-C (Mi et al., 2000). Furthermore, velocity of weight gain during childhood and catch-up obesity in low-birth-weight Asian Indian babies has been reported to be important for adult-onset hyperglycemia and cardiovascular risk factors (Sachdev et al., 2005). Whether low birth weight, childhood catch-up obesity, or increased velocity of weight gain within the normal weight range in childhood are independent factors or additive in causation of insulin resistance and the syndrome X has not been investigated. It has prompted the concept that the syndrome X originates *in utero* and that at this time key metabolic activities may get modulated, even though the exact role of nutritional and genetic factors has not been clearly elucidated. There is preliminary evidence that programming of hormonal systems in response to an adverse fetal environment may play an important role. It is speculated that alterations in neuroendocrine responses to stress, in particular adrenocortical and sympathoadrenal responses, are associated with small size at birth, which may have influence on plasma glucose, lipid concentrations, and blood pressure. These concepts and preliminary data appear interesting but lack confirmatory evidence. Furthermore, the role of micronutrient deficiencies during the perinatal period in development of chronic diseases later in life, although suggested, remains to be conclusively defined (Yajnik et al., 2008). Finally, preventive feeding of pre-pregnant and pregnant women may actually exacerbate the risk of obesity in Asian Indian neonates who have low muscle mass and excess subcutaneous adipose (Yajnik et al., 2002; Yajnik et al., 2003).

Prevalence of obesity and the syndrome X has shown a rapid rise in developing countries in the past few decades and has led to increased risk of CVD and consequent morbidity and mortality. Because both undernutrition and overnutrition are seen simultaneously in developing countries, the double burden of diseases makes the situation more difficult. The various factors responsible for increasing NCDs are rapid nutrition transition, rural-to-urban migration, increasingly sedentary occupations and lifestyle, and maternal-fetal factors. Both genetic and environmental factors seem to contribute to it; however, the role of environment seems to be predominant. Health interventions required to prevent or reduce the morbidity/mortality need to be addressed in both children and adults. Interventions should be aimed at increasing the physical activity along with healthier food patterns and health education. Successful community based intervention programs have been reported in developed countries, and a similar approach is required in developing countries. Reports of interventional programs in China and India, especially directed toward children, have shown encouraging results, but large-scale programs involving adults/children are required. Various other health strategies consisting of individual and community initiatives, backed up by governmental and legislative efforts, would also help in minimizing the increasing prevalence of obesity and the syndrome X in developing countries. (Misra & Khurana, 2008).

SOCIOECONOMIC FACTORS

The previously held view that people belonging to high SES are more predisposed to develop obesity in developing world is no longer tenable (Sobal & Stunkard, 1989). The burden of obesity in developing countries shifts toward the people belonging to lower SES as the country's GDP increases, probably because scarcity of food and/or physically demanding lifestyle become less common, even in people belonging to low SES after the economy improves. Pattern 5 of nutrition transition, in which nutrition and physical activity become more balanced than pattern 4, is mostly applicable to people belonging to high SES. This segment of population can afford relatively more expensive healthy foods and costly but healthy oils and avail of facilities and equipment for physical exercise and thus have far more flexibility in their choices of foods and activity patterns than those belonging to low SES. The latter class of people, although improving in economic status, continues to have low awareness of benefits of diet and physical activity and cannot afford healthier food choices (WHO, 2003). In Brazil, a steep increase in the prevalence of obesity has been seen in people belonging to low SES along with a decline in obesity among the higher-income groups (Monteiro et al., 1995; 2004; 2002). It is important to note that most people belonging to low SES and living in rural areas of the developing countries are lean. However, when these people migrate from rural areas to large metropolitan cities, they quickly acquire risk factors associated with urbanization despite remaining in the same SES as the previous habitat. Specifically they start smoking and consume alcohol, and their diets become imbalanced. Whereas some may still engage in physically intensive jobs, most of them are involved in sedentary jobs (e.g., stationary street hawkers). High prevalence rates of T2DM, obesity, insulin resistance, hypertension, atherogenic dyslipidemia, hyper-homocysteinemia and endothelial dysfunction have been reported in this intra-country rural-to-urban migrant population settled in urban slums (Misra et al., 2001, Vikram et al., 2003; Misra et al., 2001; 2002; 2002; Vikram et al., 2003; Sethi et al., 2002).

In particular, significant clustering of cardiovascular risk factors was seen in postmenopausal women living in urban slums in India (Misra et al., 2002; Wasir&Misra, 2004, Misra et al., 2001, Wasir et al., 2007). Similar findings have been noted in the urban slum population in Thailand (Sawaya et al., 1995, Bunnag et al., 1990; Prentice, 2006). Recently, increase in obesity and cardiovascular risk factors have been seen even in rural areas of some developing countries (Chow et al., 2008). It is important to note that many of so-called rural areas are no longer truly rural, and people are increasingly becoming urbanized (*in situ* urbanization) and mechanized even in locations far from cities. Interestingly, this phenomenon to some extent, also appears to be driven by the so-called 'remittance economy' (money sent home from family members who have become affluent after migration, which leads to relative affluence, even in rural farm-based communities) (Prentice, 2006).

Social stigma against obesity and obsession in some developed countries to remain lean has probably helped limit obesity to some extent. However, this psychosocial attitude toward obesity is not seen in many developing countries. Studies in African- Americans show a lack of social pressure to be thin and reduced stigma toward obesity, leading to higher levels of body satisfaction and acceptance of obesity by the individual and community (Littlewood, 2004; Flynn & Fitzgibbon, 1998; Kumanyika et al., 1993). For example, Gambian populations were reported to be more obesity tolerant (acceptance of obese body size as normal) than African-Americans and much more tolerant than white Americans (Siervo et al., 2006). The Polynesians have one of the highest prevalence rates of obesity in the world along with large body size with power, beauty, and affluence (Brewis et al., 1998), and Pima Indians, having the highest frequency of T2DM. Similarly, there is a general misconception in parents in India and other developing countries that an obese child is a healthy child, and hence, feel that it is important to feed him/her in excess (Bhardwaj et al., 2008). Furthermore, mothers in India often have traditional belief that feeding oils, *ghee* (clarified butter), and butter to child would be beneficial to growth and impart strength. Another important factor is increasing pressure on children to perform in academics often forced by parents and teachers, which leads to reluctance of child to take part in sports or any other form of physical activity. Specifically, the majority of children in India are physically inactive when they are studying in classes when major examinations are held (Bhardwaj et al., 2008). Lack of playfields at school and open spaces around home, and decreased stress on games and physical training in schools has further led to decline in physical activity in children. In some developing countries, due to increasing crimes, parents do not allow children to play outside alone. Lastly, but significantly, a steep increase in sedentary activities like television viewing and computer usage has substantially contributed to a rise in obesity in children (Bhardwaj et al., 2008).

CONCLUSION

Prevalence of obesity and the syndrome X has shown a rapid rise in developing countries in the past few decades and has led to increased risk of CVD and consequent morbidity and mortality. Because both undernutrition and overnutrition are seen simultaneously in developing countries, the double burden of diseases makes the situation more difficult. The various factors responsible for increasing NCDs are rapid nutrition transition, rural-to-urban migration, increasingly sedentary occupations and lifestyle, and maternal-fetal factors care causing differences in prevalence of Syndrome X by ethnicity and sex. Both genetic and environmental factors seem to contribute to it; however, the role of environment seems to be predominant. Health interventions required to prevent or reduce the morbidity/mortality need to be addressed in both children and adults. Interventions should be aimed at increasing the physical activity along with healthier food patterns and health education. Various health strategies consisting of individual and community initiatives, backed up by governmental and legislative efforts, are desperately needed to minimize the increasing prevalence of syndrome X in developing countries, across ethnicity.

REFERENCES

Al-Hazzaa HM, Al-Rasheedi AA. Adiposity and physical activity levels among preschool children in Jeddah, Saudi Arabia. *Saudi Med J.* 2007; 28: 766–773.

Al-Nozha MM, Al-Hazzaa HM, Arafah MR, Al-Khadra A, Al-Mazrou YY, Al-Maatouq MA, Khan NB, Al-Marzouki K, Al-Harthi SS, Abdullah M, Al-Shahid MS. Prevalence of physical activity and inactivity among Saudis aged 30–70 years. A population-based cross-sectional study. *Saudi Med J.* 2007; 28: 559–568.

Bavdekar A, Yajnik CS, Fall CH, Bapat S, Pandit AN, Deshpande V, Bhave S, Kellingray SD, Joglekar C. Insulin resistance syndrome in 8-year-old Indian children: small at birth, big at 8 years, or both? *Diabetes.* 1999; 48: 2422–2429.

Bhardwaj S, Misra A, Khurana, Gulati S, Shah P, Vikram NK. Childhood obesity in Asian Indians: a burgeoning cause of insulin resistance, diabetes and sub-clinical inflammation. *Asia Pac J Clin Nutr.* 2008; 17(Suppl 1): 172–175.

Brewis AA, McGarvey ST, Jones J, Swinburn BA. Perceptions of body size in Pacific Islanders. *Int J Obes Relat Metab Disord.* 1998; 22:185–189.

Bunnag SC, Sitthi-Amorn C, Chandraprasert S. The prevalence of obesity, risk factors and associated diseases in KlongToey slum and KlongToey government apartment houses. *Diabetes Res. Clin Pract.* 1990; 10 (Suppl 1):S81–S87.

Chow CK, Naidu S, Raju K, Raju R, Joshi R, Sullivan D, Celermajer DS, Neal BC. Significant lipid, adiposity and metabolic abnormalities amongst 4535 Indians from a developing region of rural Andhra Pradesh. *Atherosclerosis.* 2008; 196: 943–952.

Daryani A, Berglund L, Andersson A, Kocturk T, Becker W, Vessby B. Risk factors for coronary heart disease among immigrant women from Iran and Turkey, compared to women of Swedish ethnicity. *Ethn Dis.* 2005; 15: 213–220.

Das M, Pal S, Ghosh A. Prevalence of the metabolic syndrome in people of Asian Indian Origin: outcomes by definitions. *Cardiovasc J Afr.* 2011; 22: 303-305.

Deepa M, Farroq S, Datta M, Deepa R, Mohan V. Prevalence of metabolic syndrome using WHO, ATPIII and IDF definitions in Asian Indians: the Chennai Urban Rural Epidemiology Study (CURES-34). *Diab Metab Res Rev.* 2007; 23:127–134.

Eckel RH, Alberti KG, Grundy SM, et al. The metabolic syndrome. *Lancet.* 2010; 375: 181–183.

Flynn KJ, Fitzgibbon M. Body images and obesity risk among black females: a review of the literature. *Ann Behav Med.* 1998; 20: 13–24.

Food and Agriculture Organization. Globalization of food systems in developing countries: impact on food security and nutrition. *Food and Nutrition paper.* 2004. United Nations: Food and Agriculture Organization of the United Nations.

Ghosh A. Effects of socio-economic and behavioural characteristics in explaining central obesity—a study on adult Asian Indians in Calcutta, India. *Coll Antropol.* 2006; 30:265–271.

Grundy SM, Cleeman JI, Daniels SR, et al.; American Heart Association; National Heart, Lung, and Blood Institute. Diagnosis and management of the metabolic syndrome: An American Heart Association/National Heart, Lung, and Blood Institute Scientific Statement. *Circulation* 2005; 112: 2735–2752.

Grundy SM, Neeland IJ, Turer AT, Vega GL. Ethnic and Gender susceptibility to metabolic risk. *Metab Synd Relat Disord.* 2014; 12: 110-116.

Grundy SM. A constellation of complications: the metabolic syndrome. *Clin Cornerstone.* 2005; 7: 36-45.

Grundy SM. Metabolic syndrome: a multiplex cardiovascular risk factor. *J Clin Endocrinol Metab.* 2007; 92:n399-404.

Guthold R, Ono T, Strong KL, Chatterji S, Morabia A. Worldwide variability in physical inactivity a 51-country survey. *Am J Prev Med.* 2008; 34: 486–494.

Hales CN, Barker DJ. The thrifty phenotype hypothesis. *Br Med Bull.* 2001; 60: 5–20.

Harris JM, Kaufman PR, Martinez SW, Price C. *The U.S. Food Marketing System.* 2002. Washington, DC: U.S. Department of Agriculture Economic Research Service (agricultural economic report no. 811).

Hawkes C. Uneven dietary development: linking the policies and processes of globalization with the nutrition transition, obesity and diet-related chronic diseases. *Global Health.* 2006; 2: 4.

Henry CJ, Lightowler HJ, Al-Hourani HM. Physical activity and levels of inactivity in adolescent females ages 11–16 years in the United Arab Emirates. *Am J Hum Biol.* 2004; 16: 346–353.

Hoffman DJ. Obesity in developing countries: causes and implications. *Food, Nutrition and Agriculture.* 2001. A publication of the FAO food and nutrition division. Available at: ftp://ftp.fao.org/docrep/fao/003/y0600m/y0600m04.pdf. Last accessed July 2008.

Kabagambe EK, Baylin A, Campos H. Nonfatal acute myocardial infarction in Costa Rica: modifiable risk factors, population-attributable risks, and adherence to dietary guidelines. *Circulation.* 2007; 115: 1075–1081.

Kanjilal S, Shanker J, Rao VS, Khadrinarasimhaih NB, Mukherjee M, Iyengar SS, Kakkar VV. Prevalence and component analysis of metabolic syndrome: an Indian atherosclerosis research study perspective. *Vasc Hlth Risk Manag.* 2008; 4: 189–197.

Kelishadi R, Sadri G, Tavasoli AA, Kahbazi M, Roohafza HR, Sadeghi M, Khosravi A, Sabet B, Amani A, Ansari R, Alikhassy H. Cumulative prevalence of risk factors for atherosclerotic cardiovascular diseases in Iranian adolescents: IHHP-HHPC. *J Pediatr (Rio J).* 2005; 81:447–453.

Kumanyika S, Wilson JF, Guilford-Davenport M. Weight-related attitudes and behaviors of black women. *J Am Diet Assoc.* 1993; 93: 416–422.

Laxmaiah A, Nagalla B, Vijayaraghavan K, Nair M. Factors affecting prevalence of overweight among 12- to 17-year-old urban adolescents in Hyderabad, India. *Obesity* (Silver Spring). 2007; 15: 1384–1390.

Littlewood R. Commentary: globalization, culture, body image, and eating disorders. *Cult Med Psychiatry.* 2004; 28: 597–602.

Lobelo F, Pate R, Parra D, Duperly J, Pratt M. Burden of mortality associated to physical inactivity in Bogota, Colombia. *Rev Salud Publica* (Bogota). 2006; 8(Suppl 2): 28–41.

Matsudo V, Matsudo S, Andrade D, Araujo T, Andrade E, de Oliveira LC, Braggion G. Promotion of physical activity in a developing country: the Agita Sao Paulo experience. *Public Health Nutr.* 2002; 5: 253–261.

Mi J, Law C, Zhang KL, Osmond C, Stein C, Barker D. Effects of infant birthweight and maternal body mass index in pregnancy on components of the insulin resistance syndrome in China. *Ann Intern Med.* 2000; 132: 253–260.

Misra A, and Khurana L. Obesity and the metabolic syndrome in developing countries. *J Clin Endocrinol Metab.* 2008; 93: S9-S30.

Misra A, Chaudhary D, Vikram NK, Mittal V, Devi JR, Pandey RM, Khanna N, Sharma R, Peshin S. Insulin resistance and clustering of atherogenic risk factors in women belonging to low socio-economic strata in urban slums of North India. *Diabetes Res Clin Pract.* 2002; 56: 73–75.

Misra A, Khurana L, Isharwal S, Bhardwaj S South Asian diets and insulin resistance. *Br J Nutr.* 2009; 101(4): 465-73. doi: 10.1017/S0007114508073649.

Misra A, Pandey RM, Devi JR, Sharma R, Vikram NK, Khanna N. High prevalence of diabetes, obesity and dyslipidaemia in urban slum population in northern India. *Int J Obes Relat Metab Disord.* 2001; 25: 1722–1729.

Misra A, Pandey RM, Devi JR, Sharma R, Vikram NK, Khanna N. High prevalence of diabetes, obesity and dyslipidaemia in urban slum population in northern India. *Int J Obes Relat Metab Disord.* 2001; 25: 1722–1729.

Misra A, Pandey RM, Sharma R. Non-communicable diseases (diabetes, obesity and hyperlipidaemia) in urban slums. *Natl Med J India.* 2002; 15: 242–244.

Misra A, Vikram NK, Pandey RM, Dwivedi M, Ahmad FU, Luthra K, Jain K, Khanna N, Devi JR, Sharma R, Guleria R. Hyperhomocysteinemia, and low intakes of folic acid and vitamin B12 in urban North India. *Eur J Nutr.* 2002; 41: 68–77.

Monteiro CA, Conde WL, Popkin BM. The burden of disease from undernutrition and overnutrition in countries undergoing rapid nutrition transition: a view from Brazil. *Am J Public Health.* 2004; 94:433–434.

Monteiro CA, Conde WL, Popkin BM. Is obesity replacing or adding to undernutrition? Evidence from different social classes in Brazil. *Public Health Nutr.* 2002; 5: 105–112.

Monteiro CA, Mondini L, de Souza AL, Popkin BM. The nutrition transition in Brazil. *Eur J ClinNutr.* 1995; 49: 105–113.

Moore SE, Halsall I, Howarth D, Poskitt EM, Prentice AM. Glucose, insulin and lipid metabolism in rural Gambians exposed to early malnutrition. *Diabet Med.* 2001; 18: 646–653.

Mozaffari H, Nabaei B. Obesity and related risk factors. *Indian J Pediatr.* 2007; 74: 265–267.

Murray CJL, Lopez AD. *The global burden of disease.* 1996; Boston: Harvard School of Public Health.

Nelson RA, Bremer AA. Insulin resistance and metabolic syndrome in the pediatric population. *Metab Syndr Relat Disord.* 2010; 8: 1-14.

Oldridge NB. Economic burden of physical inactivity: healthcare costs associated with cardiovascular disease. *Eur J CardiovascPrevRehabil.* 2008; 15: 130–139.

Paeratakul S, Popkin BM, Keyou G, Adair LS, Stevens J. Changes in diet and physical activity affect the body mass index of Chinese adults. *Int J Obes Relat Metab Disord.* 1998; 22:424–431.

Pingali P, Khwaja Y. Westernization of Asian diets and the transformation of food systems: implications for research and policy. 2004. *Annual reports*; McDonald Corp.

Popkin BM. The nutrition transition and obesity in the developing world. *J Nutr.* 2001; 131: 871S–873S.

Popkin BM. The shift in stages of the nutrition transition in the developing world differs from past experiences! *Public Health Nutr.* 2002; 5: 205–214.

Popkin BM, Du S. Dynamics of the nutrition transition toward the animal foods sector in China and its implications: a worried perspective. *J Nutr.* 2003; 133: 3898S–3906S.

Popkin BM. Urbanization, lifestyle changes and the nutrition transition. *World Dev.* 1999; 27: 1905–1916.

Prentice AM. Intrauterine factors, adiposity, and hyperinsulinaemia. *BMJ.* 2003; 327:880–881.

Prentice AM. Early influences on human energy regulation: thrifty genotypes and thrifty phenotypes. *Physiol Behav.* 2005; 86: 640–645.

Prentice AM. The emerging epidemic of obesity in developing countries. *Int J Epidemiol.* 2006; 35: 93–99.

Prentice AM, Moore SE. Early programming of adult diseases in resource poor countries. *Arch Dis Child.* 2005; 90:429–432.

Prentice AM, Rayco-Solon P, Moore SE. Insights from the developing world: thrifty genotypes and thrifty phenotypes. *Proc Nutr Soc.* 2005; 64: 153–161.

Rosenzweig JL, Ferrannini E, Grundy SM, et al. Endocrine Society. Primary prevention of cardiovascular disease and type 2 diabetes in patients at metabolic risk: An Endocrine Society clinical practice guideline. *J Clin Endocrinol Metab.* 2008; 93: 3671–3689.

Sachdev HS, Fall CH, Osmond C, Lakshmy R, Dey Biswas SK, Leary SD, Reddy KS, Barker DJ, Bhargava SK. Anthropometric indicators of body composition in young adults: relation to size at birth and serial measurements of body mass index in childhood in the New Delhi birth cohort. *Am J Clin Nutr.* 2005; 82:456–466.

Sawaya AL, Dallal G, Solymos G, de Sousa MH, Ventura ML, Roberts SB, Sigulem DM. Obesity and malnutrition in a shantytown population in the city of Sao Paulo, Brazil. *Obes Res.* 2005; 3(Suppl 2): 107s–115s.

Sethi A, Misra A, Pandey RM, Luthra K, Devi JR, Sharma R, Khanna N, Dwivedi M, Vikram NK. Soluble inter-cellular adhesion molecule-1 in urban Asian north Indians: relationships with anthropometric and metabolic covariates. *Dis Markers.* 2002; 18: 111–120.

Sicree R, Shaw J, Zimmet P. Diabetes and impaired glucose tolerance in India. In: Gan D, ed. *Diabetes atlas.* 3rd ed. 2006. Kortrijik (Hevle), Belgium: International Diabetes Federation; 15–103.

Siervo M, Grey P, Nyan OA, Prentice AM. A pilot study on body image, attractiveness and body size in Gambians living in an urban community. *Eat Weight Disord.* 2006; 11: 100–109.

Smith C, Essop MF. Gender differences in metabolic risk factor prevalence in a South African student population. *Cardiovasc J Africa.* 2009; 20: 178-182.

Snipes K. *Mexico exporter guide: annual 2004*. GAIN reportMX4313. Washington, DC: United States Foreign Agricultural Service. 2004.

Sobal J, Stunkard AJ. Socioeconomic status and obesity: a review of the literature. *Psychol Bull.* 1989; 105: 260–275.

STOPP-T2D – Studies to Treat or Prevent Pediatric T2D. Prevalence of the metabolic syndrome among racially/ethnically diverse group of U.S. eighth-grade adolescents and associations with fasting insulin and homeostasis model assessment of Insulin Resistance levels. *Diabetes Care.* 2008; 31: 2020-2025.

Tailor AM, Peeters PH, Norat T, Vineis P, Bomaguera D. An update on the prevalence of the metabolic syndrome in children and adolescents. *Int. J Pediatr Obes*. 2010; 5: 202-213.

Tong PC, Kong AP, So WY, Yang X, Ho CS, Ma RC, et al. The usefulness of the International Diabetes Federation and the National Cholesterol Education Program's Adult Treatment Panel III definitions of the metabolic syndrome in predicting coronary heart disease in subjects with type 2 diabetes. *Diabetes Care.* 2007; 30:1206–1211.

Tudor-Locke C, Ainsworth BE, Adair LS, Du S, Lee N, Popkin BM. Cross-sectional comparison of physical activity and inactivity patterns in Chinese and Filipino youth. *Child Care Health Dev*. 2007; 33:5 9–66.

Vega GL, Barlow CE, Grundy SM. Prevalence of the metabolic syndrome as influenced by the measure of obesity employed. *Am J Cardiol.* 2010; 105: 1306–1312.

Victor RG, Haley RW, Willett DL, et al.; Dallas Heart Study Investigators. The Dallas Heart Study: A population-based probability sample for the multidisciplinary study of ethnic differences in cardiovascular health. *Am J Cardiol.* 2004; 93: 1473–1480.

Vikram NK, Pandev RM, Sharma R, Misra A. Hyperhomocysteinemia in healthy Asian Indians. *Am J Hematol.* 2003; 72: 151–152.

Wasir JS, Misra A, Vikram NK, Pandey RM, Gupta R. Comparison of definitions of the metabolic syndrome in adult Asian Indians. *J Assoc Physicians India.* 2008; 56: 158–164.

Wasir JS, Misra A, Vikram NK, Pandey RM, Luthra K. C-reactive protein, obesity, and insulin resistance in postmenopausal women in urban slums of North India. *Diabetes and metabolic syndrome: Clin Res Rev*. 2007; 1: 83–89.

Wasir JS, Misra A. The metabolic syndrome in Asian Indians: the impact of nutritional and socio-economic transition in India. *Metab Syndr Relat Disord.* 2004; 2: 14–23.

Wild S, Roglic G, Green A, Sicree R, King H. Global prevalence of diabetes: estimates for the year 2000 and projections for 2030. *Diabetes Care.* 2004; 27: 1047–1053.

World Health Organization 2003. Diet, nutrition and the prevention of chronic diseases. *World Health Organ Tech Rep Ser* 916: i-viii, 1–149, back cover.

World Health Organization 1998 *The World Health Report: life in the 21st century: a vision for all.* Geneva: World Health Organization.

World Health Organization 1999 *The World Health Report: making a Difference.* Geneva: World Health Organization.

World Health Organization 2002 *Diet, physical activity and health* (documents A55/16 and A55/16 Corr. 1). Geneva: World Health Organization.

World Health Organization. *Background. 2008*; Available at: http://www.who.int/nutrition/topics/2_background/en/index.html.

Yajnik CS, Deshpande SS, Jackson AA, Refsum H, Rao S, Fisher DJ, Bhat DS, Naik SS, Coyaji KJ, Joglekar CV, Joshi N, Lubree HG, Deshpande VU, Rege SS, Fall CH. Vitamin B(12) and folate concentrations during pregnancy and insulin resistance in the offspring: the Pune Maternal Nutrition Study. *Diabetologia.* 2008; 51: 29–38.

Yajnik CS, Fall CH, Coyaji KJ, Hirve SS, Rao S, Barker DJ, Joglekar C, Kellingray S. Neonatal anthropometry: the thin-fat Indian baby. The

Pune Maternal Nutrition Study. *Int J ObesRelatMetabDisord.* 2003; 27: 173–180.

Yajnik CS, Lubree HG, Rege SS, Naik SS, Deshpande JA, Deshpande SS, Joglekar CV, Yudkin JS. Adiposity and hyperinsulinemia in Indians are present at birth. *J Clin Endocrinol Metab.* 2002; 87: 5575–5580.

Zabetian A, Hadaegh F, Azizi F. Prevalence of metabolic syndrome in Iranian adult population, concordance between the IDF with the ATP-III and the WHO definitions. *Diab Res ClinPrac.* 2007; 77: 251–257.

Zimmet PZ, Alberti KG, Shaw JE. Mainstreaming the metabolic syndrome: a definitive definition. *Med J Aust.* 2005; 183: 175-176.

In: Ethnicity and Syndrome X
Editors: M. Das and K. Bose
ISBN: 978-1-53618-042-8
© 2020 Nova Science Publishers, Inc.

Chapter 2

TRANSNATIONAL MIGRATION AS A RISK FACTOR FOR SYNDROME X

Sylvia Kirchengast*
Department of Evolutionary Anthropology,
University of Vienna, Vienna, Austria

INTRODUCTION

Since the Neolithic transition more than 12,000 years ago, infectious diseases have been the main causes of morbidity and mortality in *Homo sapiens* (Larsen 1995). This situation changed in the course of the nineteenth and twentieth century as advances in medical research, in particular in bacteriology, and improvements in hygiene, medical care, but also the introduction of vaccines and antibiotics reduced the prevalence of infectious diseases and associated mortality markedly. Consequently, the successful conquest of many of the old infectious diseases during the so-called third epidemiologic transition, resulted in a dramatic rise of the prevalence of non-communicable diseases (NCDs) (Omran 1983). In other words, the ages of

* Corresponding Author's Email: sylvia.kirchengast@univie.ac.at.

pestilence and famine, typical of preindustrial societies, were followed by the age of degenerative and man-made diseases (Omran 1983). Although, without any doubt, infectious diseases have not completely disappeared and not all infections are curable today, so-called non-communicable diseases – also named civilization diseases or western diseases, are the major causes of health impairments, reduced health related quality of life and death in high income countries but also increasingly in middle- and low-income countries (Barrett et al. 1998). Typical non-communicable diseases are cardiovascular diseases, such as hypertension, heart attacks, stroke, metabolic diseases such as diabetes or hypertriglyceridemia, cancers, chronic respiratory diseases but also chronic inflammatory diseases such as allergies or autoimmune diseases (Danaei et al. 2009). According to the World Health Organization (WHO), non-communicable diseases (NCDs) are responsible for the death of about 41 million people each year, equivalent to 71% of all deaths globally (WHO 2019).

Beside cancer, the most prominent symptom complex of NCDs is the so-called metabolic syndrome or syndrome X, which is a cluster of biological factors characterized by central obesity, high waist to hip ratio, dyslipidemia, hypertension, and type 2 diabetes mellitus (Nolan et al. 2017). The link between syndrome X and an increased risk of multiple chronic diseases, such as cardiovascular disease, arthritis, chronic kidney disease, and several types of cancer and an early death have been reported for many decades (Saklayen 2018).

In order to prevent such diseases, risk factors have to be identified. Despite of a genetic disposition, there is no doubt, that the main causes of non-communicable diseases are life style factors. Consequently, health and disease patterns are highly influenced by environmental and social factors. In the present study, the impact of migration and cultural change on the development of syndrome X associated symptoms, in particular hypertension, obesity and diabetes type 2, is analyzed.

DEFINITION OF SYNDROME X

Several criteria and definitions have been used to describe syndrome X. Today, there is a consensus that a combination of three or more of the following components must be present: obesity, large waist circumference, elevated triglyceride levels, low HDL-cholesterol, hypertension, and elevated fasting blood glucose (Alberti et al., 2005). Consequently, syndrome X represents a clustering of different metabolic abnormalities and can be described as a combination of obesity, hypertension, diabetes type 2 and elevated lipid levels. Therefore, syndrome x is not a single disease, but a symptom complex and a constellation of cardiovascular disease risk factors. According to the International Diabetes Federation (IDF) and the WHO about 25% of the world's population suffer from syndrome X with increased prevalence in advanced ages (O'Neill & O'Driscoll, 2015), however, this estimate varies widely due to the age, ethnicity, and gender of the population studied.

OBESITY, DIABETES TYPE II AND HYPERTENSION

As pointed out above, the main symptoms of syndrome x are obesity, diabetes type II and hypertension which are clearly interrelated. Obesity is without any doubt a major risk factor of developing type II diabetes, but also increases the risk of some other metabolic diseases such as hypertension, dyslipidemia, coronary heart disease, pancreatitis, osteoarthritis or some forms of cancer such as breast cancer or colon cancer (Wang et al. 2011). Consequently, obesity is not only a symptom of syndrome X it is also a major risk factors of other symptoms typical of syndrome X (Kulie et al. 2011). The strong association between obesity and several diseases resulted in the following definition of obesity: Obesity is defined as a state of increased body weight, in particular increased adipose tissue, of sufficient magnitude to produce numerous adverse health consequences (Hossain et al. 2007; Ford & Mokdad 2008). For an appropriate determination of obesity commonly the body mass index (BMI) based on body weight and height (kilograms per square meter) and waist circumference, which is an indicator of central obesity, are used (WHO 1995). According to the World Health Organization, overweight is defined as a BMI above 25.00kg/m^2, while a BMI above 30.00kg/m^2 is an indicator of obesity. A BMI above 40.00kg/m^2 is interpreted as morbid obesity (WHO 1995). These cut offs are used for adult populations. Since subadult individuals are still growing, and the growth patterns differ according to sex, the definition of weight status among subadults represents a special problem. Consequently, BMI percentiles for each separate sex and age class are commonly used for the determination of overweight and obesity among children and adolescents (Lasserre et al. 2007). During the last few decades the worldwide prevalence of obesity increased dramatically (Han et al. 2010). Therefore, excess body weight and in particular obesity belong to the most serious public health challenges of the 21st century.

In 2008, for the first time in the long history of *Homo sapiens*, the number of obese people on earth exceeded the number of people suffering from starvation and undernourishment (FAO 2015). In 2014, 39% men and 40% of women aged 18+ were overweight (BMI $\geq$ 25 kg/m^2) and 11% of men and 15% of women were obese (BMI $\geq$ 30 kg/m^2). This means that more than 1.9 billion adults, 18 years and older, are overweight. Of these over 600 million correspond to the definition of obesity (WHO 2016).

Obesity is significantly linked to numerous chronic diseases, in particular to diabetes type II. Diabetes type II is characterized by chronic hyperglycemia because the target cells are unable to use the insulin effectively even if the pancreas produces it (WHO 2016). Consequently, type II diabetes is caused by the body´s ineffective use of insulin, e.g., insulin resistance. Blood glucose levels increase dramatically and may lead to the damage and dysfunction of the beta cells of the pancreas, nephropathy, retinopathy, diabetic cataracts and the damage of blood vessels (Lieberman 2003). Typical symptoms of type II diabetes are frequent urination, hunger, thirst and weight loss (Lieberman 2003).

The prevalence rates of obesity and diabetes type II are changing rapidly (WHO 2016). During the twentieth century obesity and type II diabetes were mainly found in western affluent societies. Consequently, "diabesity" was seen as a "disease of affluence". At the beginning of the 21st century however, obesity but especially diabetes type II, have become increasingly common in low- and middle-income countries (Ramachandran 2004, Hu 2011). Since 1980 the prevalence of diabetes has doubled from 4.7% to 8.5% worldwide. While in 1980 worldwide 108 million people suffered from diabetes, this was true of 422 people in 2014 (WHO 2016). More than 90% of these 422 million adults who were suffering from diabetes worldwide were affected by type II diabetes, too. This dramatic increase is mainly due to general population growth and the fact that life expectancy increased markedly during the last four decades. Prevalence rates increased in particular in low income regions such as Africa where the prevalence rates doubled from 3.1% to 7.1%. and so-called threshold countries such as India and China, or in the Eastern Mediterranean region where the prevalence rates increased from 5.9% to 13.7%. In Europe in contrast, the rates increased from 5.3% to 7.3% only. As pointed out above diabetes mellitus is no longer a disease of affluence, it is now increasingly common in poor societies (Ramachandran 2004). The largest absolute numbers of affected people are found in South Asia, East Asia and the Pacific Region (Ramachandran 2004, Joswitt 2014). These three regions account for more than 50% of people affected by diabetes worldwide (WHO 2016).

The third symptom of syndrome X considered in this paper is hypertension or with other words elevated blood pressure. Hypertension is commonly defined as a systolic blood pressure above 140 mmHg and/or the diastolic blood pressure above ≥90 mmHg. Elevated blood pressure is a serious medical condition that significantly increases the risks of heart, brain, kidney and other diseases Furthermore, high blood pressure is one of the leading causes of premature death worldwide (WHO 2019). Currently, more than 1.1 billion people worldwide suffer from hypertension, two thirds of them live in low- and middle-income countries (WHO 2019).

SYNDROME X – A DISEASE OF POVERTY?

As pointed out above, the main symptoms of syndrome X, i.e., obesity, diabetes type II and hypertension show currently high prevalence rates in low- and middle-income countries. Considering high income or western Industrialized countries, syndrome X is mainly found among people belonging to the low social strata. Consequently, a strong association between poverty and syndrome X can be assumed (Bentley et al. 2018). Syndrome X has increasingly become a disease of the poor worldwide (van den Linden et al. 2019). Additionally, another transition in syndrome X prevalence is observable with regard to the affected age groups. While in former times syndrome X was found nearly exclusively among elderly and middle-aged people, during the past few decades however, increasingly children, adolescents and young adults have been affected (Nolan et al. 2017). Consequently, we are confronted with a dramatic social dynamic in syndrome X prevalence. Considering the high rates of syndrome X and its disastrous consequences, the identification of risk factors or factors promoting syndrome has highest priority. It is well known, that beside genetics, ecological, social and cultural factors have a major impact on the development of syndrome X.

RISK FACTOR MIGRATION

A special risk factor for the development of syndrome X seems to be migration, which is defined as the movement of people from one place to another with the intentions of settling, permanently or temporarily at a new location. Migration represents an ecological, biological, social and cultural risk factor today. Despite migration to new habitats is widely found among many animal species, such as birds, fishes and mammals, and *Homo sapiens* has a long history of migration (Mascie-Taylor & Lasker 1999), current migration patterns represent an enormous social, economic and even medical problem. This is especially due to the fact, that today, people are moving in greater numbers and over greater distances than ever before (Carballo et al. 1998). The International Organization for Migration (IOM) estimated that the number of international migrants increased to 244 million globally in 2015. With other words 3.3% of the world's population migrated to other countries in 2015 (IOM 2018). Migration is triggered by push and pull factors which force people to leave their homelands and move to new areas. Beside war, economic and political instabilities, ecological factors often triggered by climactic change such as drought which cause starvation, lack of resources and poverty influence a person's decision to migrate. Furthermore, pull factors such as freedom, peace, better educational or job opportunities promote migration worldwide. The great majority of people in the world however, do not migrate across borders, much larger numbers migrate within countries, mostly from rural to urban areas. The most recent global estimate indicates that more than 740 million people had migrated within their own country of birth in 2015 (IOM 2018). People mostly try to move to better areas nearby – a behavior which was typical for more than 99% of our history when the subsistence of *Homo sapiens* was based on hunting and gathering (Prentice 2005).

Beside internal migration, since the last few years transnational and even transcontinental migration gain in importance. These increased rates of migration are mainly the result of globalization, increased political instabilities, war and civil wars and ecological disasters. Furthermore, poverty and economic inequalities force transnational and transcontinental migration. Preferred destination regions of transnational and transcontinental migration are the classical countries of immigration such as USA, Canada, Australia and the European Union.

Migration and Health

Beside social components migration has a complex effect on health and disease patterns (Uitewaal et al. 2004 a,b; Abate & Chandalia 2007; Misra & Ganda 2007). This is true of rural – urban migrations as well as of transnational and transcontinental migration. It is well documented that migration generates both economic and non-economic changes for migrants and their families and these factors have major implications for those who migrate, but also for those who are left behind and those who host migrants (Carballo et al. 1998). In case of transnational or transcontinental migration, improved health of migrants of the first generation was observed and was called "healthy migrant effect" (Adanu & Johnson 2009; Razum et al. 1998). On the other hand, migration and migrant status represent severe stress factors which have a major impact on health and disease patterns (Popkin & Urdy 1999). Once migrants have moved to their new area of settlement, they are mostly confronted with drastic changes of their everyday life which might increase stress and affect their somatic and psychic condition. Especially in case of transnational or transcontinental migration, they have to deal with new cultural patterns, foreign language, different nutritional and life style habits (Wolin et al. 2008) Furthermore, they are a minority group in the host country, often with a lower socioeconomic position (SEP) than the host population. Minority status but also a low SEP are associated with increased chronic distress and as a consequence, higher morbidity rates (Dotevall et al. 2000; Landman & Cruishank 2001; Bongard et al. 2002; Ujcic-Voortman et al. 2009). In contrast to the so called "healthy migrant effect" pointed out above, Rogler et al. (1991) pointed out that the confrontation with culture change and acculturation represents a major stress factor which might increase the risk of developing somatic and psychic diseases. This phenomenon was later called the "acculturative stress" hypothesis and widely used in mental health studies and generalized to an array of other health outcomes research with migrant populations.

Migration and Non-Communicable Diseases

Migrants are affected with many different health risks and diseases. A special health problem among migrants is the high prevalence of non-communicable diseases (Abate & Chandalia 2007, Skogberg 2014).

OBESITY AMONG MIGRANTS

Considering that obesity is a major risk factor for non-communicable diseases, the analysis of obesity rates among migrants is particularly important. Several studies demonstrated high rates of overweight and obesity among migrants, especially among women, children and adolescents (Brussard et al. 2001; Hoppichler & Lechleitner 2001; Kirchengast & Schober 2006, Kirchengast & Singh 2011, Kilaf & Kirchengast 2011). In many Central and Northern European countries immigrants from Mediterranean countries, the Near and Middle East are described as extremely vulnerable to become overweight or obese (Brussard et al. 2001; Hoppichler & Lechleitner 2001; Fredriks et al. 2005; Dijkshoorn et al. 2008; Uitewaal et al. 2004; Kirchengast & Schober 2006; Misra & Ganda 2007; Faskunger et al. 2009; Wolin et al. 2009). In a Viennese study, migrant women originating from Turkey and from India showed highly significantly higher rates of overweight and obesity than their age matched Austrian counterparts (Kilaf & Kirchengast 2011; Kirchengast & Singh 2011). A high prevalence of overweight and obesity (3.6-49.4%) is also found among immigrants from Northern Africa in Europe. The highest frequency of physically inactive or lightly active people among immigrants was observed in first-generation Sudanese and Moroccans in Amsterdam (males: 57.1%; females: 74.2%), with increasing rates in second-generation females (Toselli et al. 2014). Studies from the United States focusing on the situation of Hispanic immigrants showed similar results (Kaplan et al. 2004; Park et al. 2009). Recently, some authors claim that immigrant obesity is the result of an unhealthy assimilation and the low socioeconomic position of immigrants (Van Hook & Balisteri 2007; Faskunger et al. 2009; Park et al. 2009). Furthermore, a strong association between obesity and the length of residence in the host country was reported (Kaplan et al. 2004).

A special problem represents obesity among children with a background of migration. Childhood or adolescence obesity is generally an enormous health hazard because childhood or adolescent obesity results not only in social stigmatisation of overweight or obese children and deleterious social and economic consequences (Latner & Stunkard 2003), there are also implications for long-term health and longevity. Childhood obesity is acknowledged to be an increasingly strong predictor of adult obesity. Several studies have demonstrated that childhood obesity is one of the most important risk factors for hypertension, diabetes mellitus, or abnormal lipid levels in other words, childhood obesity promotes syndrome X in later life (Must et al. 1992). Additionally, childhood obesity increases psychic and emotional morbidity (Latner & Stunkard 2003). The longterm consequences of childhood obesity are also socioeconomic ones, obese children and adolescents complete fewer years of education, and have lower household income in adulthood, independent of familial socioeconomic status (Haas et al. 2003). As a consequence, obesity among migrant children is an additional factor contributing to an increased risk of longterm poverty, impaired health and increased mortality. Without any doubt, these fatal consequences of obesity affect not only migrant children but children with a background of migration are especially vulnerable to become obese (Haas et al. 2003, Kirchengast & Schober 2005). Obesity is largely caused by an environment that promotes excessive food intake and discourages physical activity (Hill & Peters 1998). This kind of environment is commonly called obesogenic (Lieberman 2006). The majority of migrants hope for better lives for themselves and their children and interpret energy dense food, characterized by a high amount of refined sugar and fat but also physical inactivity as a luxury lifestyle (Green et al. 2003; Hosper et al. 2007; Lawrence et al. 2007). Consequently, migrants adapted very fast to an obesogenic environment in Europe or the United States. They and their children are confronted with advertisements and opportunities to purchase food that is relatively cheap and of low nutritional quality. Therefore, immigrant obesity is often interpreted as the result of an unhealthy assimilation of immigrants (Van Hook & Balisteri 2007; Faskunger et al. 2009; Park et al. 2009)

In our Viennese project we could demonstrate that migrant children show significantly higher prevalence rates of overweight and obesity from the age of six years onwards (Kirchengast & Schober 2006).

Diabetes among Migrants

Numerous studies show clearly that migrant status increases not only the risk of obesity but also of type II diabetes (Abate & Chandalia 2007, Montesi 2016). This is true of Hispanic immigrants in the United States (Schneiderman et al. 2014) as well as of immigrants originating from Mediterranean countries or the Middle East in Central and Northern Europe (Uitewaal et al. 2004). The incidence and mortality rates for diabetes type II are much higher among migrants in comparison to their host population (Montesi et al. 2016). Studies from the United Kingdom reveal, that the prevalence of diabetes type II is around 25% among migrants from Afghanistan, Bhutan, Maledives, Nepal, and Sri Lanka. This is nearly five times higher than the host population (Montesi et al. 2016). Comparable results were found for the Netherlands where the diabetes type II is more common among migrants from Turkey, Morocco, Suriname and the Antilles (Montesi et al. 2016). In the United States, migrants originating from Mexico and Central America, but also from Asia, such as from China, India, Fillipines, Hawaii or the Pacific Islands are at an increased risk to develop diabetes type II (Montesi et al. 2016). In our Viennese study, significantly higher rates of diabetes type II among migrants from Turkey and Former Jugoslavia in comparison to age matched Austrians have been documented (Kirchengast & Schober 2006). Beside genetic factors, first of all adverse nutritional habits and physical inactivity are the main reasons for this trend (Misra et al. 2005).

Hypertension among Migrants

Hypertension or high blood pressure disproportionately affect ethnic minority groups and migrants in nearly all high-income countries (Dawson et al. 2019). In the Untied States, first of all migrants originating from Mexico and Central America, but also from Asia and Russia suffer from hypertension, a leading factor for cardiovascular disease (Commodore-

Mensah et al. 2018; Divney et al. 2019). Similar prevalence patterns are found in Canada, Australia and Europe (Bhatnagar et al. 1995, Kaplan et al. 2002). Hypertension is mainly the results of distress, obesity but also a lack of physical activity and adverse nutritional habits such as a diet characterized by a high content of sugar, fat and salt. This kind of life style is frequently found among migrants who quickly changed to an obesogenic environment but who are also confronted with low socioeconomic status and acculturation stress.

Discussion

What are the reasons for the high rates of overweight or obesity and syndrome X among migrants? From the viewpoint of Evolutionary Anthropology in the high prevalence of obesity and syndrome X associated with migration to new cultural settings, acculturation and modernization may be interpreted as a result of a maladaptation of recent *Homo sapiens* to postmodern environments. As early as 1962, James Neel proposed the thrifty gene hypothesis to partially explain the rise in type 2 diabetes and obesity in the 20th century (Neel 1962). The central premise of his theory is that natural selection has favored the ability to store and utilize energy efficiently because our ancestors went through a cycle of feast and famine. Individuals whose energy storage or utilization was increased were more likely to survive and reproduce during periods of starvation. Consequently, efficient energy storage was a beneficial adaptation. In the recent obesogenic environment however, efficient energy storage turned to be maladaptive resulting in obesity and all associated problems increasing urbanization, mechanization of jobs, improvement of transportation services, the availability of processed and fast food of high energy density, and reduced physical activity (Popkin 2003, Popkin & Gordon-Larsen 2004).

From a physiological point of view overweight and obesity are caused by an imbalance between energy intake and expenditure (Florentino 2002), but the imbalance between energy intake and expenditure is beside genetic factors mainly attributed to environments that are obesogenic (Poston II &

Foreyt 1999, Ulijaszek 2007). Today, in high-income countries an obesogenic environment is mainly found among lower socioeconomic groups, while in low- and middle-income countries the opposite is true. Many low- and middle-income countries have achieved a remarkable improvement in nutrition status in the past decades and consequently obesity rates increased (Ramachandran 2004, Yoon et al. 2006, Garg et al. 2009, Erem 2015; Hawley & McGarvey 2015). People of high socioeconomic status who had undergone a rapid transition in nutritional habits and general lifestyle are more likely to be obese. Nevertheless, the prevalence of undernourishment is still a serious problem, especially among the poor (Abdullah 2015). Consequently, obesity and all associated problems are not interpreted as health hazards but as signs of high status and wealth. This positive interpretation obesity and even associated symptoms is transferred via transnational or transcontinental migration to high-income countries. Migrants originating from low-income countries interpret an obesogenic environment in the host country as a positive sign of improved living conditions. The transition from a lifestyle typical of low-income countries to a life in a Western society is accompanied by modernization and sometimes acculturation. Both effect nutritional habits, physical activity patterns and consequently weight status (Green et al. 2003, Lawrence et al. 2007). The problem is, that migrants mostly adapt to life circumstances of people of low socioeconomic status in high-income countries and they are not worried about obesity and syndrome X. Consequently, a rapid rise in rates of obesity, and non-communicable diseases such as type II diabetes is found among people with a background of migration in many high-income countries (Wolin et al. 2008, Skogberg 2014, Dawson et al. 2019). Furthermore, it is well established that the chances of becoming obese and suffering from syndrome X are greater for women than men and for those of lower educational level and lower socioeconomic position (Van Hook & Balistreri 2007, Faskunger et al. 2009; Park et al. 2009; Skogberg 2014).

During the 1980s and the early 1990s the British epidemiologist David Barker developed a theory of prenatal programming of later life diseases based on in utero nutritional deficiencies (Barker 1999). According to Barker life course plasticity was the key to explain obesity but also syndrome X epidemic. In particular, low birth weight newborns respond to their low level of nutritional intake in early life through alterations in growth and metabolism, which increase the risk of obesity and diabetes type 2 in later life (Barker and Clarke 1997). Barker postulates that low birth weight newborns have metabolically thrifty mechanisms for fat storage and glucose sparing with reduced rates of glucose oxidation in insulin-sensitive target tissues (Barker 1999).

The so-called barker hypothesis may explain high rates of obesity and syndrome X among migrants too. Mothers of first generation-migrants may have suffered from malnutrition before and during pregnancy, and therefore the fetuses have been confronted with a stressful intrauterine environment. Consequently, their metabolism has been prepared for a shortage of energy. The migration of an affluent society and an obesogenic environment, may have disastrous consequences, in particular an increased risk to develop obesity, diabetes type II and syndrome X (Skogberg 2014). Furthermore, migrants belong mainly to the poor of the guest society and poverty is especially associated with an obesogenic environment.

Both hypotheses, the thrifty gene hypothesis as well as the thrifty phenotype hypothesis interpret the rise of syndrome X and obesity as a result of rapid environmental change, in an evolutionary or ontogenetic sense (O´Keefe et al. 2004). Migrants experience rapid environmental change as a kind of acculturation and often modernization of life style. It is well documented, that acculturation and modernization enhance obesity rates and lead to a drastic increase of the prevalence of diabetes type II and other metabolic abnormalities (Lieberman 2003). Typical examples are hunter and gather populations such as Australian Aborigines (O´Dea et al. 1993).

Migrants undergo a similar kind of modernization and acculturation but in a much faster manner.

CONCLUSION

Obesity and syndrome X, in particular hypertension and diabetes type II, are frequently found among migrants in high-income countries. The high prevalence of syndrome X among migrants maybe interpreted as a result of a dramatic mismatch between their new environment and the environment they grew up. The rapid transition to an obesogenic environment in combination with a low social and socioeconomic status but also with a lot of psychic distress enhance metabolic disturbances. Acculturation to modern lifestyles in affluent western societies represent one the one hand an important stress factor, which has a marked impact on health and disease patterns of migrants. On the other hand, the new life style characterized by physical inactivity and the consumption of high quantities of energy dense food is interpreted as a sign of new luxury life style by many migrants. Both contribute to the high prevalence rates of syndrome X among migrants in Western high-income countries.

References

Abate N, Chandalia M 2007. Ethnicity, type 2 diabetes and migrant Asian Indians. *Ind J Med Res* 125: 251-258.

Abdullah A. 2015. The Double Burden of Undernutrition and Over-nutrition in Developing Countries: An Update. *Curr Obes Rep* 4: 337-349.

Adanu RMK, Johnson TRB. 2009. Migration and women's health. *Int J Gynecol Obstet* 106: 179-181.

Alberti KG, Zimmet P, Shaw J 2005. The metabolic syndrome - a new worldwide definition. *Lancet* 3666: 1059-1062.

Barrett R, Kuzawa CW, McDade T, Armelagos GJ (1998) Emerging and re-emerging infectious diseases: The third epidemiologic transition. *Ann Rev Anthropol* 27: 247-271.

Barker DJP, Clark PM. 1997. Fetal undernutrition and disease in later life. *Rev Reprod* 2: 105-112.

Barker DJP. 1999. Fetal origins of type 2 diabetes mellitus. *Ann Int Med* 130: 322-324.

Bentley RA, Ormerod P, Ruck DJ 2018. Recent origin and evolution of obesity-income correlation across the United States. *Palgrave Commun* 4: 146 doi: 10.1057/s41599-018-0201

Bhatnagar D, Anand IS, Durrington PN, Patel DJ, Wander GS, Mackness MI, Creed F, Tomenson B, Chandrashekhar Y, Winterbotham M, Britt RP, Keil JE, Sutton GC. 1995. Coronary risk factors in people from Indian subcontinent living in West London and their siblings in India. *The Lancet* 345: 405-409.

Björntorp P. 1988. The associations between obesity, adipose tissue and disease. *Acta Med Scand* 723: 121-134.

Bongard S, Pogge SF, Arslaner H, Rohrmann S, Hodapp V. 2002. Acculturation and cardiovascular reactivity of second-generation Turkish migrants in Germany. *J Psychosomatic Res* 53: 795-803.

Brussard JH, Erp-Baart MA van, Brants HAM, Hulshof KFAM, Löwik MRH. 2001. Nutrition and health among migrants in the Netherlands. *Pub Health Nut* 4: 659-664.

Carballo M, Divino JJ, Zeric D. 1998. Migration and health in the European Union. *Trop Med Int Health.* 12: 936-44.

Commodore-Mensah Y, Selvin E, Aboagye J, Turkson RA, Li X, Himmelfarb CD, Ahima RS, Cooper LA. 2018. Hypertension, overweight/obesity and diabetes in the United States: an analysis of the 2010-2016 national health Interview Survey. *BMC Public Health* 218: 773-783.

Danaei G, Ding EL, Mozaffarian D, Taylor B, Rehm J, Murray CJ, Ezzati M 2009. The preventable causes of death in the United States: comparative risk assessment of dietary, lifestyle and metabolic risk factors. *PLoS Med* 6: e1000058.

Dawson AZ, Walker RJ, Gregory C, Egede LE. 2019. Relationship between social determinants of health and systolic blood pressure in United States immigrants. *Int H Cardiol Hypertension* 2: 1-8.

Dijkshoorn H, Nierkens V, Nicolaou M. 2008. Risk groups for overweight and obesity among Turkish and Moroccan migrants in The Netherlands. *Public Health* 122: 625- 630.

Dinc G, Eser E, Saatli GL, Cihan UA, Oral A, Baydur H, Ozcan C. 2006. The relationship between obesity and health related quality of life of women in a Turkish city with a high prevalence of obesity. *Asia Pacific J Clin Nutr* 15: 508-515.

Divney AA, Echeverria SE, Thorpe LE, Trinh-Shevrin C, Islam NS. 2019. Hypertension prevalence jointly influenced by acculturation and gender. in US immigrant groups. *Am J Hypertension* 32: 104-111.

Dotevall A, Rosengren A, Lappas G, Wilhelmsen L. 2000. Does immigration contribute to decreasing CHD incidence? Coronary risk factors among immigrants in Göteborg, Sweden. *J Internal Med* 247: 331-339.

Erem C. 2015. Prevalence of Overweight and Obesity in Turkey. *Int J Clin Metab Endocrine* 8: 38-41.

FAO. 2015. *The state of food insecurity in the world* 2015. Food and Agriculture Organization of the United Nations. Rome.

Faskunger J, Eriksson U, Johansson SE, Sundquist K, Sundquist J. 2009. Risk of obesity in immigrants compared with Swedes in two deprived neighborhoods. *Public Health* 9: 304-312.

Ford ES, Mokdad AH 2008. Epidemiology of obesity in the Western hemisphere. *J Clin Endocrinol Metab* 93: S1-S8.

Fredriks AM, van Buuren S, Hira Sing RA, Wit JM, Verloove-Vanhorick SP. 2005. Alarming prevalence of overweight and obesity for children of Turkish, Moroccan and Dutch origin in The Netherlands according to international standards. *Acta Paediatrica* 94: 496-498.

Garg C, Khan SA, Ansari SH, Garg M 2009. Prevalence of obesity in Indian women. *Obes Rev* 11: 105-108.

Green J, Waters E, Haikerwal A, O`Neill CO, Raman S, Booth ML, Gibbons K. 2003. Social, cultural and environmental influences on child activity and eating in Australian migrant communities. *Child Care Health Develop* 29: 441-448.

Haas JS, Lee LB, Kaplan CP, Sonneborn D, Phillips KA, Liang SY. 2003. The association of race, socioeconomic status and health insurance status with the prevalence of overweight among children and adolescents. *Am J Public Health* 93: 2105-2110.

Han JC, Lawlor DA, Kimm SY 2010. Childhood obesity *The Lancet* 375: 1737-1748.

Hawley NL, McGarvey ST. 2015. Obesity and diabetes in Pacific islanders: the current burden and the need for urgent action. *Curr Diab Rep* 15: 19-29.

Hoppichler F, Lechleitner M. 2001. Counseling programs and the outcome of gestational diabetes in Austrian and Mediterranean Turkish women. *Pat Edu Counsel* 45: 271-274.

Hosper K, Klazinga NS, Stronks K. 2007. Acculturation does not necessarily lead to increased physical activity during leisure time: a cross-sectional study among Turkish young people in the Netherlands. *Public Health* 7: 230-239.

Hossain P, Kawar B, El Nahas M. 2007. Obesity and diabetes in the developing world – a growing challenge. *New Eng J Med* 356: 213-215.

Hu FB. 2011. Globalization of diabetes. *Diabetes Care* 34: 1249-1257.

IOM 2018. *World migration reports*. /www.iom.int.

Jowitt LM. 2014. Ethnicity and type 2 diabetes in Pacific Island adults in New Zealand. *Int J Diab Clin Res* 1:1-5.

Kaplan MS, Chang C, Newson JT, McFarland BH. 2002. Acculturation status and hypertension among Asian immigrants in Canada. *J Epidemiol Comm Health* 56: 455-456.

Kaplan MS, Huguet N, Newsom JT, McFarland BH. 2004. The association between length of residence and obesity among Hispanic immigrants. *Am J Prev Med* 27: 323-326.

Kilaf E, Kirchengast S. 2011. Obesity among Turkish migrant women in Vienna, Austria. *J Life Sci* 3: 107-116.

Kirchengast S, Schober E. 2006. To be an immigrant: a risk factor for developing overweight and obesity during childhood and adolescence. *J biosoc Sci* 38: 695-705.

Kirchengast S, Singh M. 2011. Obesity prevalence and nutritional habits among Indian women: a comparison between Punjabi women living in India and Punjabi migrants in Vienna, Austria. *Anthrop Anz* 68: 239-251.

Kulie T, Slattengren A, Redner J, Counts H, Ehglash A, Schrager S. 2011. Obesity and women´s health: an evidence-based review. *J Am Board Fam Med* 24: 75-85.

Lasserre AM, Chiolero A, Paccaud F, Bovert P. 2007. World-wide trends in childhood obesity. *Swiss Med Weekly* 137: 157-158.

Landman J, Cruickshank JK. 2001. A review of ethnicity, health and nutrition related diseases in relation to migration in the United Kingdom. *Public Health Nutr* 4: 647-657.

Larsen C. 1995. Biological changes in human populations with agriculture. *Annu Rev Anthropol* 24: 185-213.

Latner JD, Stunkard AJ. 2003. Getting worse: the stigmatisation of obese children. *Obes Res* 11: 452-456.

Lawrence JM, Devlin E, Macaskill S, Kelly M, Chinouya M, Raats MM, Barton KL, Wrieden WL, Shepherd R. 2007. Factors that affect the food choices made by girls and young women, from minority ethnic groups, living in the UK. *J Hum Nutr Diet* 20: 311-319.

Lieberman LS. 2003. Dietary, evolutionary and modernizing influences on the prevalence of type 2 diabetes. *Annu Rev Nutr* 23: 345-377.

Lieberman LS. 2006. Evolutionary and anthropological perspectives on optimal foraging in obesogenic environments. *Appetite* 47: 3-9.

Mascie-Taylor CGN, Lasker GW 1999. *Biological aspects of human migration.* Cambridge University Press.

Misra A, Ganda OP. 2007. Migration and its impact on adiposity and type 2 diabetes. *Nutrition* 23: 696-708.

Misra KB, Endemann SW, Ayer M. 2005. Leisure time activity and metabolic syndrome in Asian Indian immigrants in northern California. *Ethnicity & Disease* 15; 627-634.

Montesi L, Caletti MT, Marchesini G. 2016. Diabetes in migrants and ethnic minorities in a changing world. *World J Diabetes* 7: 34-44.

Must A, Jaques PF, Dallal GE, Bajema CJ, Dietz WH. 1992. Long term morbidity and mortality of overweight adolescents: a follow up of the Harvard Growth Study of 1922 to 1935. *New England J Med* 327: 1350-1355.

Neel V. 1962. Diabetes mellitus: a thrifty genotype rendered detrimental by progress? *Am J Hum Genet* 14: 353-362.

Nolan PB, Carrick-Ranson G, Stinear JW, Reading SA, Dalleck LC. 2017. Prevalence of metabolic syndrome and metabolic syndrome components in young adults: A pooled analysis. *Preventive Med Reports* 7: 211–215.

O´Dea K, Hopper J, Patel M, Traimedes K, Kubisch D. 1993. Obesity. Diabetes, and hyperlipidemia in a Central Australian Aboriginal community with a long history of acculturation. *Diabetes Care* 16: 1004-1010.

O´Keefe Jr JH, Cordain L. 2004. Cardio-vascular disease resulting from Diet and Lifestyle at odds with our Paleolithic genome: how to become a 21rst century hunter-gatherer. *Mayo Clinic Proceed* 79: 101-108.

Omran A. 1983. The epidemiologic transition theory: a preliminary update. *J Trop Ped* 29: 305-316.

O´Neill S, O´Droscoll L. 2015. Metabolic syndrome: a closer look at the growing epidemic and its associated pathologies. *Obes Rev* 16: 1-12.

Park J, Myers D, Kao D, Min SH. 2009. Immigrant obesity and unhealthy assimilation: Alternative estimates of convergence or divergence, 1995-2005. *Soc Sci Med* 69: 1625-1633.

Pentice AM. 2005. Starvation in humans: Evolutionary background and contemporary implications. *Mech Age Develop* 126: 976-981.

Popkin BM. 2001. The nutrition transition and obesity in the developing world. *J Nutr* 131: 871-873.

Popkin BM, Gordon-Larsen P. 2004. The nutrition transition: worldwide obesity dynamics and their determinants. *Int J Obes* 28: 52-59.

Popkin BM, Udry JR. 1998. Adolescent obesity increases significantly in second and third generation U.S. Immigrants: The National Longitudinal study of adolescent health. *J Nutr* 128: 701-706.

Poston II WSC, Foreyt JP. 1999. Obesity is an environmental issue. *Atherosclerosis* 146: 201-209.

Ramachandran A. 2004. Diabetes and obesity – the Indian angle. *Indian J Med Res* 120: 437-439.

Razum O, Zeeb H, Akgün HS, Yilmaz S. 1998. Low overall mortality of Turkish residents in Germany persists and extends into second generation: merely a healthy migrant effect? *Trop Med Int Health* 3: 297–303.

Rogler LH, Cortes DE, Malgady RG. 1991. Acculturation and mental health status among Hispanics: Convergence and new directions for research. *Am Psychol* 46: 585–597.

Saklayen MG. 2018. The Global Epidemic of the Metabolic Syndrome. *Curr Hypertension Reports* 20: 12-20.

Schneiderman N, Llabre M, Cowie CC, Barnhart J, Carnethon M, Gallo LC, Giachello AL, Heiss G, Kaplan RC, LaVange LM, Teng Y, Villa-Caballero L, Avilés-Santa ML. 2014. Prevalence of Diabetes Among Hispanics/Latinos From Diverse Backgrounds: The Hispanic Community Health Study/Study of Latinos (HCHS/SOL) *Diabetes Care* 37: 2233-2239.

Skogberg N. 2014. Association between socioeconomic position and health behavior with metabolic syndrome among migrants of Russian, Somali and Kurdish origin in Finland. *Eur J Public Health* 24: 256.

Toselli S, Gualdi-Russo E, Boulos DNK, Anwar WA, Lakhoua C, Jaouadi I, Khyatti M, Hemminki K. 2014. Prevalence of overweight and obesity in adults from North Africa. *Eur J Public Health* 24: 31-39.

Uitewaal PJM, Manna DR, Bruijnzeels MA, Hoes AW, Thomas S. 2004. Prevalence of type 2 diabetes mellitus, other cardiovascular risk factors, and cardiovascular disease in Turkish and Moroccan immigrants in North West Europe: a systematic review. *Prev Med* 39: 1068-1076.

Uitewaal PJM, Goudswaard AN, Ubnik-Veltmaat LJ, Bruijnzeels MA, Hoes AW, Siep T. 2004. Cardiovascular risk factors in Turkish immigrants with type 2 diabetes mellitus: Comparison with Dutch patients. *Eur J Epidemiol* 19: 923-929.

Ujcic-Voortman JK, Schram MT, Jacobs-van der Bruggen MA, Verhoeff AP, Baan CA. 2009. Diabetes prevalence and risk factors among ethnic minorities. *Eur J Pub Health* 19: 511-515.

Ulijaszek SJ. 2007. Obesity: a disorder of convenience. *Obes Reviews* 8: 183-187.

Van der Linden EL, Meeks K, Beune E, de-Graft Aikins A, Addo J, Owusu-Dabo E, Mockenhaupt FP, Bahendeka S, Danquah I, Schulze MB, Spranger J, Klipstein-Grobusch K, Tetteh Appiah L, Smeeth L, Stronks K, Agyemang C. 2019. The prevalence of metabolic syndrome among

Ghanaian migrants and their homeland counterparts: the Research on Obesity and type 2 Diabetes among African Migrants (RODAM) study. *Eur J Public Health.* 0: 1–8.

Van Hook J, Balistreri KS 2007. Immigrant generation, socioeconomic status and economic development of countries of origin: A longitudinal study of body mass index among children. *Soc Sci Med* 65: 976-989.

Wang Y, Lobstein T. 2006. Worldwide trends in childhood overweight and obesity *Int J Ped Obes* 1: 11-25.

Wang Y, McPherson K, Marsh T, Gortmaker SL, Brown M. 2011. Health and economic burden of the projected obesity trends in the USA and the UK. *The Lancet* 378: 815-825.

Withrow D, Alter DA 2011. The economic burden of obesity worldwide: a systematic review of the direct costs of obesity. *Obes Rev* 12: 131-141

WHO. 1995. *Physical status the use and interpretation of anthropometry.* WHO technical Reports Series 854, Geneva 1995.

WHO. 2016. *Global Report on Diabetes*, Geneva.

Wolin KY, Colangelo LA, Chiu BCH, Gapstur SM. 2008. Obesity and immigration among Latina women. *J Immigrant Minority Health* 11: 428-431.

Yoon KH, Lee JH, Kim JW, Cho JH, Ko SH, Zimmet P, Son HY. 2006. Epidemic obesity and type 2 diabetes in Asia. *The Lancet* 368: 1681-1682.

In: Ethnicity and Syndrome X
Editors: M. Das and K. Bose
ISBN: 978-1-53618-042-8
© 2020 Nova Science Publishers, Inc.

Chapter 3

ETHNIC DIVERSITIES AND RISK FACTORS WITH SYNDROME X IN SOUTH AFRICA

Yackoob Kassim Seedat*
Emeritus Professor, University of KwaZulu-Natal,
Durban, South Africa

INTRODUCTION

> "Lord! We know what we are but we know not what we be."
> Ophelia in Hamlet - William Shakespeare

South Africa is a large country with a surface area of just over 1.2 million square kilometres situated on the southern tip of Africa. Its population is about 57 million and is growing at the rate of 2.5% a year. The percentage of the population is 76.2% Black, 13.3% White. 8.6% "mixed" and 2.6% Indian. South Africa is a middle-income country with a gross national product of US $2,560 per person in 1991. Give US dollar = 14.6

* Corresponding Author's Email: seedaty1@gmail.com.

Rands. The unemployment rate is 27.6% among blacks. There are gross income inequalities in South Africa, 51% of the annual incomes go to the richest 10% of households whilst under 4% goes to the poorest 40%.

One of the important characteristics of the South African economy is the inequality between the racial groups Urban Foundation (1991), World Bank (1993). The Gini index is the highest in the world. Fallon and da Silva estimate that in 1987 whites earned 9.5 times per person than blacks. This has shown little improvement in post-apartheid South Africa which occurred in 1994. The majority of whites live in cities which have a modern infrastructure and have well-funded schools and modern hospitals. Most black urban localities have much poorer services and large numbers live in shanty towns. The rural black population has poor access to public services. (Fallon and da Silva (1994).

The high-income earners include the majority of whites. Most live in their own homes or rented accommodation, in well-serviced parts of the cities. The majority are members of medical aid schemes. About 6.7 million are either members of these schemes or purchase private health insurance. The number of people in the high-income group is between 7 and 8 million or between 17% and 20% of the population. The government defines households as poor if their annual income is below the annual datum line. This was about 9,500 Rands per household in 1993. Du Toit and Falkana (1993) estimate that about half of South Africa is poor by this definition. The conditions of life in these areas are similar to poor areas in other parts of sub-Saharan Africa, where people find it difficult to obtain clean water, there is inadequate disposal of human wastes, literacy levels are low and a large proportion of children are malnourished. The highest levels of poverty are in the inner and outer periphery where over 60% of the population have incomes below the household subsistence level, and where the population is mainly black. The rapid migration of blacks to the metropolitan centres has led to a growing problem of urban poverty.

Syndrome X

This Syndrome X has been given many names. Recently WHO has termed it as a Metabolic Syndrome. It is a clustering of cardiovascular risk factors (Table). Insulin resistance is a characteristic feature of Asian Indians. It is a probable cause of coronary artery disease (CAD). There is a clustering of risk factors. Diabetes mellitus is mainly due to insulin resistance and increases the risk of CAD by 2 – 4-fold.

Components of the metabolic syndrome (Syndrome X)

- Insulin resistance/hyperinsulinemia
- Central obesity
- Hypertension
- Dyslipidemia
  - Increased plasma triglycerides
  - increased serum cholesterol
  - Decreased Hdl cholesterol
- Endothelial dysfunction
- Microalbuminuria
- Inflammatory markers
  - C-reactive protein
- Hyperuricemia
- Polycystic ovary syndrome

(A Ramachandran, 2005)

Hypertension

A World Health Organisation (WHO) analysis shows that the prevalence of hypertension in developing countries varies from 1% in some African countries to > 30% in Brazil. (Nissenen 1988) Hypertension is common in the urban black population of Africa. Our age-corrected prevalence studies of Durban, show that in the adult black population of Durban, hypertension (WHO criteria) was highest in urban Zulus (25%), intermediate in whites (17.2%) and lowest (14%) in the Indian population. (Seedat, 1983).

The mean systolic blood pressures (SBP) and diastolic blood pressures are lower than in the West Indies, Nigeria and African Americans. The difference in mean arterial pressure between African American and urban Zulus is probably due to African Americans having been accultured for 300 years, whereas urban blacks have been accultured only since the turn of the century.

Hypertension develops at an earlier age in African Americans than in whites (Comstock, 1957) (Weiss and Prusmack, 1938), in South Africa. We have found that females between the ages of 35 and 40 years have a higher prevalence than males. The higher prevalence of hypertension in blacks under the age of 40 years, probably explains the younger age groups of hypertensive patients at autopsy (Isaacson, 1977).

The determinant factors among blacks are genetic factors, personal characteristics autonomic nervous system functions, cardiac functions and various environmental factors. Black hypertensive subjects have a higher plasma sodium and lower plasma potassium concentration than normotensive subjects. (Weissberg et al., 1987). In the South African black populations red cell magnesium and serum plasma potassium, magnesium and calcium were found to be significantly lower than in black hypertensive subjects (Touyz, 1987). There were racial differences in potassium transport suggesting that blacks have a limited capacity to exchange intracellular sodium for intracellular potassium and a higher percentage of this exchange is dependent upon obtain sensitive mechanism. We found that lymphocyte intracellular sodium was significantly higher than in hypertensive blacks compared to normotensive blacks. Black subjects excrete sodium loads more slowly and have a markedly lower urinary kallikrein excretion. Plasma renin activity in lower urinary kallikrein excretion. Plasma renin activity (PRA) is lower in blacks and does not increase in response to sodium and volume depletion (Hoosen et al., 1990).

Insulin resistance is a characteristic feature of Asian Indians, although most of them have lean body mass by Western standards. (Mckeigue et al., 1991). Obesity is an important cause of hypertension especially in urban black females of sub-Saharan Africa. It forms an important component of Syndrome X. (Mckeigue et al., 1991. It is more common in urban compared to rural Zulus (black) females. We have found important social factors that predispose to hypertension in our urban black population. They are socio-economic status, married people with more children, and those who spend more time going to work and live in more deprived or less favoured townships. Urban hypertensive blacks have higher incidence of insomnia, anxiety, cigarette smoking, lower educational status, greater number of children not working, lack of recreation and sports and overcrowding in homes. (Seedat et al., 1982).

The clinical pattern of hypertension in hospitalised patients is a rapid course with death frequently from cerebral haemorrhages or thrombosis. Uraemia may frequently occur. Malignant hypertension is an important cause or morbidity and mortality among urban black South Africans. Hypertension accounts for 16% of all hospitalised patients and 35% of blacks receiving treatment for end stage renal failure. Acute and partially reversible renal failure occurs in 20% of patients with malignant hypertension who require dialysis. This important sub-group is characterised by youth, female preponderance and fulminant presentation. Short-term peritoneal dialysis and effective control blood pressure and effective control of blood pressure may result in satisfactory return of renal function. Renovascular hypertension and hypertension due to fibromuscular hyperplasia in adult blacks is uncommon. In our experience primary arteritis of the aorta and renal arteries is an important cause of renovascular hypertension. (Seedat YK, 1988).

Coronary Heart Disease

Coronary heart disease (CHD) in prosperous Western populations rose markedly in the 1940's, peaked between 1970 and 1975 and then fell variably by about 50% in the USA and Australia. In South Africa, in all population groups other than blacks, CHD rose similarly, with whites and Asians attaining very high rates. However, from 1978 to 1989, the total death rate among white males (per 100 000) fell from 1002 to 631 (37%) and the CHD mortality from 312 to 139 (56%). Rates for Asians were 1306 to 1130 (14%) and 355 to 226 (36%) respectively and for the "mixed" group 1691 to 1392 (18%) and 171 to 110 (36%). For blacks the data are unreliable but it appears that total mortality rates remained unchanged and CHD rates are low. Knowledge of the rise and fall in CHD remain incomplete. (Walker et al., 1993.)

Historically, coronary artherosclerosis was a disease of antiquity, evident in the thickening and calcification of coronary arteries in Egyptian mummies dating from about 100 BC. In about 800 BC, Indian physicians, who knew of the circulation of the blood, described anginal pain as a "sense of constriction in the praecordium, stitching pain and sensations of churners, bursting or rubbing". Coronary heart disease is a major problem in migrant Indians throughout the world. Our study in the Indian community of Durban shows that there were important risk factors leading to CHD. (Seedat et al., 1990), (Seedat et al., 1991). The most important risk factors were hypercholesterolaemia, hypertriglyceridemia, diabetes mellitus and smoking and in females, diabetes, hypercholesterolaemia and hypertriglyceridemia. The minor risk factors were hyperuricaemia, sedentary occupations, obesity in women and a positive family of CHD. A study of the major risk factors leading to CHD showed that 45.5% (age and sex adjusted) had at least one major risk factor (level A) and 61.9% had lower (level B) risk levels. Diabetes was strongly associated with a family history of CHD. There was a strong association of hypertension with triglyceridaemia, obesity, hypercholesterolaemia suggesting an underlying state of insulin resistance. This has been postulated by McKeigue, 1991, in the South Asian population of London. The concept of insulin resistance is an interesting one to explain the high incidence of CHD in migrant incidence throughout the world. In 48.2% (age and sex adjusted) of the total group, electrocardiogram (ECG) abnormalities were found that could be coded.

In our study of risk factors leading to CHD in the white community we found that the important risk factors were hypercholesterolaemia, hypertension and smoking. The minor risk factors were obesity, hypertriglyceridaemia, hyperuricaemia, a sedentary occupation and a history of CHD in the immediate family. ECG abnormalities denoting CHD were present in 17% of the subjects. A study of the major risk factors showed that 35.1% (age and sex adjusted) had lower risk levels (level B). When the combinations of risk factors were taken into account, 15.2% and 28% had two major risk factors, one each at levels A and B respectively. On average the percentage of men and women with one risk factor or more increased with age. A protective high – density lipoprotein / total cholesterol (HDL/TC) ratio ≥ 20% was present in 53.5% of the respondents. Because of the severe nature of CHD in the Indian and white population, an intensive programme for the primary prevention of CHD risk factors should be instituted. (Seedat YK et al., 1994). Our study of CHD in the blacks looked at the missing links as to why blacks do not develop CHD to the same extent as whites or Indians. In black males, smoking and hypertension, and among black females, hypertension and obesity have merged as important risk factors. In our study the mean serum cholesterol level for all ages and both sexes fell within the normal range. Protective HDL/TC ratios were observed in about 50% of subjects. A high HDL/TC ratio, which protects against CHD has also been found in a study of blacks in the Cape Peninsula. This differs from our study of Indians and whites in Durban in which the HDL/TC ratio ≥ 20% was 62.7% and 53.5% respectively. When two risk factors co-existed, the combination of hypertension and smoking was most frequent in males (11%) and the combination of hypercholesterolaemia and hypertension most prevalent in females (3.5%). Our study showed that hypercholesterolaemia did not feature as an important risk factor in combination with other risk factors. Roberts feels that the only absolute, unequivocal, independent, atherosclerotic risk factor leading to CHD is elevated serum total cholesterol (TC) or a raised level of low density lipoprotein (LDL) cholesterol. The other 9 or the 10 risk factors leading to atherosclerosis which have been listed by the National Cholesterol Education Program on Detection, Evaluation and Treatment of High Blood Cholesterol in adults are cholesterol dependent factors. It is probable that the low incidence of CHD in blacks is due to the presence of low TC and high HDL cholesterol in adults. The other risk factors for CHD present in our black population VIZ. hypertension and cigarette smoking in males and hypertension and obesity in females, appear to be conditional on the presence of a nutritional-metabolic milieu characterised by a high intake of saturated fat and the presence of hyperlipidaemia. The risk factors work synergistically rather than additively, and the duration of exposure to risk factors, perhaps particularly during childhood, is very important. (Seedat YK et al., 1992).

The incidence of CHD in blacks in South Africa will rise again once changes in dietary patterns lead to increased lipid abnormalities. Since the data on the high prevalence of hypertension in blacks were first published there has been no mass campaign on the prevention, screening and treatment of hypertension in South Africa. Thus we have probably lost 10-15 years in the control of hypertension and its complications. A policy of primordial prevention of CHD by control of risk factors and preemptive action to prevent their spread in the population has been recommended to underdeveloped nations by a World Health Organisation Expert Committee. The primary prevention of hypertension, especially in urban populations, is the ideal approach to the primordial prevention of cardiovascular diseases, of which CHD is a small component.

CONCLUSION

There has been no other country besides South Africa in which races have been segregated so distinctly and in which socio-economic differences have rested so clearly on colour. Since 1994 major constitutional changes in the country have taken place and this is changing the lifestyle of the population. The differences in disease patterns in South Africa are mainly due to the varying patterns in the racial groups regarding their lifestyle and socio-economic status. The inequalities in the health structure are being addressed and it will lead to an emphasis on primary health care. The control of hypertension and other risk factors leading to CHD like cigarette smoking and hyperlipidaemia remain major challenges for the state and the community at large – a therapeutic challenge for the future. Other diseases like the HIV/AIDS epidemic and tuberculosis will compete for a greater share of the finance within a limited health budget.

REFERENCES

Central Statistical Service 1990a: 1.4, 3.26-3.34. *South African Statistics* 1990 Pretoria: Government Printer.

Cornstock GW. An epidemiologic study of blood pressure levels in a biracial community in the Southern United States. *Am. J. Hyg.* 1957; 65: 271-315.

Du Toit J, Falkena H (1993). *The Structure of the South African Economy* Halfway House: Southern Book Publishers (for ABSA Bank).

Fallon P, da Silva L (1994). *South Africa: Economic Performance and Policies Discussion Paper 7.* Johannesburg: The World Bank, Southern African Development.

Hoosen S, Seedat YK, Bhigjhee AI, Neerahoo RM. A study of urinary sodium and potassium excretion rates among urban sodium and potassium excretion rates among urban and rural Zulus and Indians. *J. Hypertension* 1985; 68: 351-358.

Hoosen S, Seedat YK, Bhigjhee AI. A study of urinary and intracellular sodium and potassium, renin, aldosterone and hypertension in blacks and Indians in Natal. *Cardiovasc Drugs Ther* 1990; 104: 124-132.

McKeigue PM, Shar B, Mannot MG. Relation of central obesity and insulin resistance with high diabetes prevalence and cardiovascular risk in South Asians. *Lancet* 1991; 337: 382-386.

Nissensen Al B~thig S, Granroth H, Lopez AD. Hypertension in developing countries. *World Health Stat. Q.*1988; 41: 141-154.

Roberts WC. Atherosclerotic risk factors – are there ten or is there only one. *Am. J. Cardiol.* 1989; 64:552-554.

Seedat YK, Mayet FGH, Gouws E. Risk factors for coronary heart disease in the white community in Durban. *S. Afr. Med. J.* (1994); 87: 257-262.

Seedat YK, Mayet FGH, Joubert G. Insulin resistance and hypertension: a study of coronary heart disease in the Durban Indian. *Coronary Heart Disease* 1991; 2: 1089-1091.

Seedat YK, Mayet FGH, Khan S, Somers SR, Joubert G. Risk factors for coronary heart disease in the Indians of Durban. *S. Afr. Med. J.* 1990; 78: 447-454.

Seedat YK, Mayet PGH, Latiff GH, Joubert G. Risk factors and coronary heart disease in Durban blacks – the missing links. *S. Afr. Med. J.* 1992; 82: 251-256.

Seedat YK, Pillay N, Marcoyannopoulou-Fojas H. Myocardial infection in the African hypertensive patient. *Am.*

Seedat YK, Seedat MA, Hackland DBT. Biosocial factors and hypertension in urban and rural Zulus. *S. Afr. Med. J.* 1982; 61: 999-1002.

Seedat YK, Seedat MA, Hackland DBT. Prevalence of hypertension in the urban and rural Zulu. *J. Epidemiol. Commun. Health* 1982; 36: 256-261.

Seedat YK. Primary arteritis of the aorta and its branches. *S. Afr. Med. J.*1988; 74: 438-443.

Seedat YK. Race, environment and blood pressure: The South African experience. *J. Hypertension* 1983; 1: 7-12.

Seedat YK. The clinical pattern of hypertension in the South African black population. A study of 1000 patients. *N.Z. Med. J.* 1974; 79: 946-951.

Seedat YK. Varying responses to hypotensive agents in different racial groups: black versus white differences. *J. Hypertens.* 1989; 7: 515-518.

The Expert Panel. Report of the National Cholesterol Education Program Expert Panel on detection, evaluation and treatment of high blood cholesterol in adults. *Arch Intern Med* 1988; 148:36-69.

Urban Foundation (1991). *Population Trends: Demographic Projection Model Johannesburg: Urban Foundation.*

Walker ARP, Adam A, Kustner HGV. Changes in total death rate and in ischaemic heart disease in interethnic South African populations, 1878-1989. *.S Afr. Med. J.* 1993; 83: 602-605.

Weiss MM, Prusmack JJ. Essential hypertension in the Negro. *Am. Med. Sci.* 1938; 195: 510-516.

In: Ethnicity and Syndrome X
Editors: M. Das and K. Bose
ISBN: 978-1-53618-042-8
© 2020 Nova Science Publishers, Inc.

Chapter 4

A COMPARATIVE STUDY ON NUTRITIONAL STATUS AMONG TRIBAL AND NON-TRIBAL MOTHERS IN RAJSHAHI DISTRICT BANGLADESH: A CROSS-SECTIONAL STUDY

Md. Masud Rana[1,*], Md. Reazul Karim[1], Md. Rafiqul Islam[1], Premananda Bharati[2] and Md. Golam Hossain[3]

[1]Department of Population Science and Human Resource Development, University of Rajshahi, Rajshahi, Bangladesh
[2]BiologicalAnthropology Unit, Indian Statistical Institute, Kolkata
[3]Department of Statistics, University of Rajshahi, Rajshahi, Bangladesh

ABSTRACT

Nutritional assessment in the community is very essential for accurate planning and implementation of intervention programmes to reduce morbidity and mortality associated with under-nutrition. The objective of

---

* Corresponding Author's Email: masud.raj82@gmail.com.

this study was to investigate the current nutritional status among mothers and compare in nutritional status between tribal and non-tribal in Rajshahi district, Bangladesh.

It was a cross sectional and household level study. A multi-indicator survey designed was prepared to explore a number of different and diverse issues related to health and nutrition among mothers. The proposed areas for this study were the catchment areas of CCs in Rajshahi district, Bangladesh. All rural areas of this district were included in catchment areas of CCs. The data was collected from the field survey conducted from October to December, 2016. Chi-square test was used in this study to examine the association between tribal and non-tribal mothers. A total number of 540 were considered as sample for investigation of nutritional status among tribal (57, 10.46%) and non-tribal (488, 89.54%) mothers in the rural area of Rajshahi district, Bangladesh. It was noted that out of total number of mothers, 17.8% and 19.1% mothers were under nourished and over nourished respectively.

This study determined the prevalence and associated factors of malnutrition among tribal and non-tribal mothers in the rural area of Rajshahi district, Bangladesh and compared in nutritional status between tribal and non-tribal mothers in the same region. Consequently, this study recommended to Bangladeshi Government should provide social safety net program for mothers, especially for tribal mothers.

Keywords: Chi-square test, malnutrition, Tribal Rajshahi district, Bangladesh

INTRODUCTION

Nutrition is the science that interprets the interaction of nutrients and other substances in food in relation to maintenance, growth, reproduction, health, and disease of an organism (Arai, 2014). It is the intake of healthy food and balanced diet, considered in relation to the body's dietary needs and it makes easier to choice the better food for health (WHO, 2017). Human body dependants upon intake of adequate quality of food and it required variety of foods to meet for essential nutrients, and the value of a various diet has long been recognized (Arimond and Ruel, 2004). The high nutrients demands of children and their mother for growth and reproduction in developing countries is risk because consumption of low-quality, common monotonous diets and socio-cultural phenomena (Arimond et al., 2010). Globally, approximately 13% of women were estimated to be undernourished, and 38% of all pregnant women suffered from anaemia (Stevens, et al., 2013). Furthermore, micronutrient deficiencies in particular vitamin A, zinc, iodine, and iron are estimated to affect more than 2 billion people globally, with adverse effects that include premature death, poor health, blindness, stunting, reduced cognitive development, and low productive capacity (Bhutta, et al., 2013). Poor nutritional status is a major public health problem throughout the developing countries (Black et al. 2008). The preschool children (aged 6-59 months) are malnourished if their height-for-age and weight-for-height, weight-for-age, is below minus two standard deviations (SDs) from the median of the World Health Organization (WHO) Child Growth Standards (WHO, 2006). Worldwide, it was estimated that one in every three preschool children is malnourished. In 2016, an estimation of 41 million children under-five years of age were underweight, 155 million were stunted and 52 million were wasted (UNICEF, 2017). Child undernutrition is estimated to underline 3.1 million deaths annually, equivalent to 45% of all child deaths are linked to malnutrition in low and middle income countries (Black et al., 2013). In South-Asia, estimates show that 37% of children younger than five years of age are stunted and 46% are underweight (Stevens et al., 2012). The underlying determinants of malnutrition in South Asia are manifold and in some respect multiplicative (Ikeda et al., 2013). Maternal malnutrition is a key contributor to poor fetal growth, low birth weight (LBW) and infant morbidity and mortality and can cause long-term, irreversible and detrimental cognitive, motor and health impairments. Undernutrition in females may occur during childhood, adolescence and pregnancy, and has a cumulative adverse impact on the birth weight of future babies (Victora et al., 2008). Maternal health during pregnancy and exclusive breast-feeding and while caring for a child is a useful predictor of pregnancy outcomes and the subsequent nutritional status of a child. Malnourished mothers can contribute the likelihood of giving birth to children with anemia or LBW (Karim et al., 2016).

Most of the study were took place in children. To the best of our knowledge this type of study has not been conducted yet in Bangladesh. Special attention should be paid to tribal mother considering their potential influence on their family and their contribution to the nation's workforce in near future in a particular nation. Due to their unique role in near future in the society, it is important to investigate the current nutritional status among mothers and compare in nutritional status between tribal and non-tribal. The objective of this study was to investigate the current nutritional status among mothers and compare in nutritional status between tribal and non-tribal in Rajshahi district, Bangladesh.

MATERIAL AND METHODS

Study Design and Population

This was a cross sectional and household level study. A multi-indicator survey designed was prepared to explore a number of different and diverse issues related to health and nutrition among mothers. The proposed areas for this study were the catchment areas of CCs in Rajshahi district, Bangladesh. All rural areas of this district were included in catchment areas of CCs. Rajshahi district located in the north-western part of Bangladesh and separated from India by a branch of Ganges River (Padma branch). The total area of the district is 2425.37 km^2 and the population are 2,699,688 (BSS, 2011) and consists of 9 Upazilas, 71 Unions and 1,587 villages. There are 232 functional CCs in Rajshahi district. The northwest of Rajshahi lies between the elevated and undulating Barind region; to the south is the high, well-drained Padma Valley; and a swampy depression drains the land in the immediate vicinity of the city (Uddin et al., 2014). Rajshahi is the one of the highest poverty zones in Bangladesh (BBS, 2009). Around 2.3% ethnic minority representative whom is most deprived population (BBS, 2011).

Sample Size Determination

The following mathematical formula was used to determine the sample size for this study:

$$n = \frac{N}{1 + Nd^2}$$

where, n = required sample size, N= household size (in here 2,71,302), d = marginal error (we considered, $d = 0.05$), 95% confidence level (CI) had been considered (Rana et al., 2015). The formula provided that the significant sample size was 399 for this study. Initially, we considered 576 households, unfortunately 31 households head did not agree to provide their information, and consequently 545 households were considered for this study.

DATA COLLECTION

The data was collected from the field survey conducted from October to December, 2016. All selected samples were interviewed by an expert researchers group. Socio-economic, demographic, anthropometric and behavioral factors were collected from our selected subjects.

Sample Procedures

Multistage sampling technique was utilized to select samples covering all the population from all upazilas of Rajshahi district. There are 9 upazilas of Rajshahi district and in these upazilas 232 CCs are running. In the first stage, 2 CCs had been selected from each upazila by simple random sampling. A total of 18 (9x2) CCs were selected. In the second stage, 2 villages had been selected from each selected CC catchments areas by random sampling, total of 36 (18x2) villages were selected. In the third stage, 16 households had been selected from each selected village by random sampling those had at least one mother having at least one tribal and non tribal mothers. The tribal and non tribal mothers were identified by their identification number (holding number or listing). All information was got from respective UP. If there was more than one tribal and non tribal mother in same household, one mother had been selected by lottery. If selected mother had more than one preschool child, last born children was considered. Since 31 individuals did not agree to participate in our study, consequently, a total of 545 tribal and non-tribal mothers were considered as a sample in the present study.

Outcome Variables

Nutritional status of mothers was the outcome variable for this study. Mothers' nutritional status was measured by their body mass index (BMI), and it was classified into three classes such as (i) under nutrition (BMI < 18.5 kg/m^2), (ii) normal (18.5 kg/m$^2 \leq$ BM < 25 kg/m^2) and over nutrition (BMI ≥ 25 kg/m^2). The BMI was defined as the weight in kilograms (kg) divided by the square of the height in metres (m).

Independent Variables

We included socioeconomic and demographic factors as independentvariables. We classified education into three groups: education was classified based on the formal education system in Bangladesh: Illiterate (0 years), primary education (1–5 years), secondary and higher (6 yearsor more). Age at first marriage in years, place of residence was categorized as <18 years, 18-24 years and ≥25 years. Age at first child birth was categorized as 20 years, 20-25 years and ≥26 years. Subjects average monthly expenditure in BDT was categorized as <5,000 in BDT, 5,000-9,999 in BDT and or ≥10,000 in BDT. Socio-economic status was categorized as hardcore poor, poor and middle-rich.

Questionnaire

A semi-structured questionnaire was duly pre-tested for collecting data from the respondents. First of all, a mini data collection was done from different study fields to observe whether there was any lacking or draw back in the questionnaire. After proper modification questionnaire was finalized and made ready for data collection. Completed questionnaires were checked on a daily basis for accuracy and completeness in recoding of responses.

Statistical Analysis

Editing and coding were done before data entry. Data were entered and analyzed using SPSS (IBM version 20). The presence of abnormal point in data set, can affect the interpretation of results. The present author checked the outlier of the data set. In this study quantitative variables and socio economic were explained descriptive analysis. Chi-square (χ^2)-test was used in this study to examine the association between tribal and non tribal mothers' nutritional status and other selected variables (independent variables). Significance associated variables were considered as independent factors for further statistical analysis.

Ethics Approval and Consent to Participate

We submitted out study protocol to ethics committee of Institute of Biological Science (IBSc) University of Rajshahi, Bangladesh. The committee provided a clearance letter for collecting data from our selected samples. Written consent was obtained from each participant.

RESULTS

A total number of 540 were considered as sample for investigation of nutritional status among tribal (57, 10.46%) and non-tribal (488, 89.54%) mothers in the rural area of Rajshahi district, Bangladesh. Our samples were representative for both tribal (Santal) and non-tribal according to the population size in Rajshahi district. In the present study, we also compared in nutritional status between tribal and tribal mothers in the same region.

Table 1 shows the socio-economic and demographic profile among tribal and nontribal mothers. It was observed that more than 50% tribal mothers were illiterate while only 9.5% non-tribal mothers were illiterate. More than three times higher number of non-trial mothers (68.7%) were secondary and higher educated than that of tribal mothers (19.3%). Slight more number of non-tribal mothers (40.6%) got marriage in their early age (age <18 years) than that of tribal mothers (36.8%). It was looked that the early child bearing mothers among non-tribal mothers (50.9%) were higher than that of tribal (43.9%). Socio-economic status of tribal and non-tribal mothers were measured by their monthly family income, and it was noted that more than 75% and only 15.7% tribal and non-tribal mothers were living in poorest family, respectively. On the other hand, 43.1% non-tribal and only 7.0% tribal mothers lived in middle or rich family. As a results, non-tribal mothers expended more money than that of tribal mothers (Table 1).

It was noted that out of total number of mothers, 17.8% and 19.1% mothers were under nourished and over nourished respectively (Table 2). When we compared tribal with non-tribal mothers, it was found that more number of tribal mothers (38.6%) were under nourished than non-tribal mothers (16.2%), but the number of over nourished among non-tribal mothers (20.3%) was higher than that of tribal mothers (16.2%). Chi-square test demonstrated that the association between mothers' nutritional status and ethnic groups was significant ($p < 0.01$). The number of over nourished mothers increased with increasing their education level, however the association between these two factors was not significant ($p > 0.05$). Again, it was found that the number of over nourished mothers increased with increasing their monthly expenditure, the association between these two factors was significant ($p < 0.01$). The number of under nourished mothers decreased and the number over nourished mothers increased with increasing their socio-economic status, the association between mothers' nutritional status and their socio-economic status was significant ($p < 0.01$). In this study, we did not find significantly association between mothers' age at first marriage ($p > 0.05$) and age at first child birth with their nutritional status (Table 2).

Table 1. Socio-economic and demographic profile of tribal and non-tribal mothers in Rajshahi district

Variables	Tribal, N(%) 57(10.46)	Non-tribal, N(%) 488(89.54)
Education level, N(%)		
Illiterate,76(14.1)	30(52.6)	46(9.5)
Primary,121(22.4)	16(28.1)	105(21.7)
Secondary and higher 343(63.5)	11(19.3)	332(68.7)
Age at first marriage in years, N(%)		
<18,217(40.2)	21(36.8)	196(40.6)
18-24, 314(58.1)	34(59.6)	280(58.0)
≥25,09(1.7)	02(3.5)	07(1.4)
Age at first child birth, N(%)		
<20,271(50.2)	25(43.9)	246(50.9)
20-25,244(45.2)	28(49.1)	216(44.7)
≥26,25(4.6)	04(7.0)	21(4.3)
Average monthly expenditure in BDT, N (%)		
<5,000 BDT,158(29.3)	42(73.7)	109(22.6)
5,000-9,999 BDT,269(49.8)	11(19.3)	220(45.5)
≥10,000 BDT,113(20.9)	04(7.0)	154(31.9)
Socio-economic status, N (%)		
Hardcore poor,119(22.0)	43(75.4)	76(15.7)
Poor, 209(38.7)	10(17.5)	199(41.2)
Middle-rich,212(39.3)	04(7.0)	208(43.1)

Table 2. Association between mother's nutritional status and socio-economic and demographic factors

Variables	Nutritional status			p-value
	Under nutrition 96(17.8%)	Healthy nutrition 341(63.1%)	Over nutrition 103(19.1%)	
Ethnic status, N(%)				0.004
Tribal,57(10.6)	22(38.6)	31(54.4)	04(7.0)	
Non- tribal,483(89.4)	74(16.2)	310(63.5)	99(20.3)	
Education level, N(%)				0.573
Illiterate,76(14.1)	17(22.4)	45(59.2)	14(18.4)	
Primary,121(22.4)	18(14.9)	83(68.6)	20(16.5)	
Secondary and higher 343(63.5)	61(17.8)	213(62.1)	69(20.1)	
Age at first marriage in years, N(%)				0.460
<18,217(40.2)	43(18.9)	137(64.1)	37(17.1)	
18-49, 323(59.8)	53(16.4)	204(63.2)	66(20.4)	
Age at first child birth, N(%)				0.104
<20,271(50.2)	55(20.3)	172(63.5)	44(16.2)	
20-25,269(49.8)	41(15.3)	169(62.8)	59(21.9)	
Average monthly expenditure in BDT, N(%)				0.009
<5,000 BDT,158(29.3)	42(26.6)	91(57.6)	25(15.8)	
5,000-9,999 BDT,269(49.8)	36(13.4)	181(67.3)	52(19.3)	
≥10,000 BDT,113(20.9)	18(15.9)	69(61.1)	26(23.0)	
Socio-economic status, N(%)				0.004
Hardcore poor,119(22.0)	34(28.6)	68(57.1)	17(14.3)	
Poor, 209(38.7)	26(12.4)	143(68.4)	40(19.2)	
Middle-rich,212(39.3)	36(17.0)	130(61.3)	46(21.7)	

DISCUSSION

All mothers living in the rural area of Rajshahi district was considered as population in this study, from this population we selected 545 tribal (10.46%) and non-tribal (89.54%) samples for investigation their nutritional status with compared between two groups considering their some socio-economic and demographic factors. Association between these factors and mothers' nutritional status was determined by Chi-square test.

In this study, we found that more number of tribal mothers were illiterate than non-tribal mothers living in the same region in Rajshahi district. In Santal (Tribal) community, the family is dominated by female and most of the tribal female work in field as farmer. they are not interested to go school, one of the most important reasons for low number of Santal female are uneducated compared to non-tribal mothers. The household quintile index and female education level have been increasing in Bangladesh during the last two decades (NIPORT, 2014). Bangladesh Government and Non-government organization has been working for improving economic condition and education among tribal community in this country; consequently their economic condition and education level have been changed. The organizations are trying to make awareness about well being and disease among tribal population in Bangladesh, they have planed to minimize the difference between tribal and non-tribal people in this country. We observed that non-tribal mothers got marriage and delivered their first baby earlier than tribal mothers. In Bangladesh more than 90% people are following Muslim religion but tribal people follows other religion, comparatively low educated rural Muslim parents want to make marriage their girls earlier as a results non-tribal female become mothers earlier than tribal. Now, in Bangladesh, below 18 years old for female marriage is illegal, and the education level among females has been increasing, consequently the average age at first marriage among Bangladeshi women has been increasing during two decades (NIPORT, 2014).

In this present study, we investigated the nutritional status about tribal and non tribal mothers, in the rural area of Rajshahi district, Bangladesh. We found that 17.8% mothers living in Rajshahi rural area was under nourished which was less than our national figure, the nationally representative data showed that 31% women aged 15-49 years had been suffering from under nutrition (NIPORT, 2014). The over nourished mothers (19.1%) in Rajshahi rural was less than that of our nationally representative women (24%) (NIPORT, 2014). The under nourished mothers in Bangladesh has been decreasing during the last 15 years, in the same duration it was found that the over nourished mothers increased rapidly due to increasing the household wealth quintile in this country (NIPORT, 2014).

We compared in nutritional status between tribal and non-tribal mothers. It was observed that the number of under nourished tribal mothers was larger than that of non-tribal mothers, but near to three times higher the number of over nourished mothers among non-tribal than tribal mothers. In this study, we found that the household wealth quintile among tribal community was less than non-tribal in the same region. It was one of the major causes for the differentiating in nutritional status between tribal and non-tribal mothers, because household wealth quintile that is, economic condition is directly related to the nutritional status in a particular population. Bangladesh Demographic and Health Survey, 2014 data demonstrated that more number of poor mothers in Bangladesh suffering from under nutrition than mothers living in rich family, but the more number of rich mothers was suffering from over nutrition (NIPORT, 2014).

Still, there are some problems among tribal community; people are not interested to take modern treatment usually most of the time tribal people take treatment from traditional healer, kabiraj and their religious leader. They hesitate to mix with non tribal community. Other problem, women in tribal community work in field like men in non-tribal community, they do not get sufficient foods as a results most of the tribal mothers suffering from chronic energy deficiency.

Most of the tribal people were land less, their monthly income is low and monthly average expenditure also very low, as results tribal mothers were suffering under nutrition than non tribal mothers, same results were found in Madagascar population (Ravaoarisoa, 2018). In this study a supplementary observation most of tribal people were hardcore poor, they live hand to mouth. Most of the tribal people were under privilege in their community, society even country health and all type of socio economic hard core poor mother tribal mothers were suffering under nutrition than non tribal mothers, same results were found in Madagascar population (Ravaoarisoa, 2018).

Strength of the Study

The main strength of this study was to first time investigated in nutritional status among Santal (tribal) mothers in Rajshahi rural area. This was the first time to compare in nutritional status between tribal and non-tribal mothers living in same region. The standardized questionnaire format was carefully developed to ascertain accurate information from the participants, the interviewers were trained, and the fieldwork was monitored by the principal investigator of this study. The data contained information on potential confounding factors, with a low proportion of missing information. The study can be generalized to other types of tribal and non tribal mothers in Bangladesh because tribal and non tribal mothers from all over the country have similar level of characteristics in Bangladesh except hill tracts.

Limitation of the Study

First of all, the study was based on a cross-sectional data from the household level and all information collected from mothers. We didn't cross check at health facilities level (upazila health complex, union health and family welfare center and community clinic). Secondly, this study didn't take into account some important variables that affect the nutritional status of children such as dietary aspects and did any biochemical test at individual level. The data has been collect from the rural area only, not considered the urban area. Therefore it is difficult to conclude the universal results from this study.

Conclusion

In this study, we determined the prevalence and associated factors of malnutrition among tribal and non-tribal mothers in the rural area of

Rajshahi district, Bangladesh. Also, we compared in nutritional status between tribal and non-tribal mothers in the same region. Our selected statistical model provided that 17.8% and 19.1% mothers in Rajshahi district were suffering from under nutrition and over nutrition respectively. Among the under nourished mothers, it was found that 38.6% and 16.2% tribal and non-tribal mothers were suffering from under nutrition respectively. The number of over nourished tribal and non-tribal mothers was 7% and 20.3% respectively. It was found that some modifiable factors were associated with nutritional status of mothers in Rajshahi district.

Consequently, Bangladesh Government should provide social safety net program for mothers, especially for tribal mothers. Health care authorities should arrange intervention programs to make sure so that health information and health education may be easily accessible for the tribal mothers. The services should be fully ensured for the underprivileged people by the health service providers. The health service providers should ensure the comprehensive health services for the tribal mothers including health education on correct nutritional practice. The Government and Non-government donor agencies and researchers may accept the findings of this study to improve the nutritional statuses of tribal mothers in Bangladesh.

Competing Interests

The authors declare that they have no competing interests.

Funding Source

None.

Authors' Contributions

MGH designed the study. MMR collected data and conducted the data analysis and wrote the manuscript. MRK, MRI and PB made critical revisions of the manuscript. All authors read and approved the final version of the manuscript.

ACKNOWLEDGMENTS

The authors gratefully acknowledge the authority of community clinic of Rajshahi, District, Bangladesh for giving permission to take data from community clinic catchment area. We also acknowledge DASCOH Foundation and Swiss Red Cross for helps to collected data from community clinic.

REFERENCES

Arai, T. (2014). The development of animal nutrition and metabolism and the challenges of our time. *Journal Frontiers in Veterinary Science*, 1(23):1. doi:10.3389/fvets.2014.00023.

Arimond, M., & Ruel, M. T. (2004). Dietary diversity is associated with child nutritional status: evidence from 11 demographic and health surveys. *The Journal of Nutrition*, 134(10):2579-2585.

Arimond, M., Wiesmann, D., Becquey, E., Carriquiry, A., Daniels, M. C., Deitchler, M., Martin-Prevel, Y. (2010). Simple Food Group Diversity Indicators Predict Micronutrient Adequacy of Women's Diets in 5 Diverse, Resource-Poor Settings–. *The Journal of Nutrition*, *140*(11): 2059S-2069S.

Bhutta, Z. A., Das, J. K., Rizvi, A., Gaffey, M. F., Walker, N., Horton, S., Black, R. E. (2013). Evidence-based interventions for improvement of maternal and child nutrition: what can be done and at what cost? *The Lancet*, 382(9890):452-477.

Black, R. E., Allen, L. H., Bhutta, Z. A., Caulfield, L. E., De Onis, M., Ezzati, M., Group, C. U. S. (2008). Maternal and child undernutrition:

global and regional exposures and health consequences. *The Lancet*, 371(9608):243-260.

BBS, WFP and World Bank. (2009). Poverty Maps of Bangladesh 2010. *Bangladesh Bureau of Statistics* and World Food Programme and World Bank, Dhaka. Available at: https://www.wfp.org/sites/default/files/Poverty%20Map%202010.

BBS. (2011). Population and Housing Census 2011. *Bangladesh Bureau of Statistics.* Statistics and Informatics Division, Ministry of Planning. Government of the People's Republic of Bangladesh.

Ikeda, N., Irie, Y., & Shibuya, K. (2013). Determinants of reduced child stunting in Cambodia: analysis of pooled data from three Demographic and Health Surveys. *Bulletin of the World Health Organization, 91*(5):341-349.

Karim, M. R., Mondal, M. N. I., Rana, M. M., Karmaker, H., Bharati, P., & Hossain, M. G. (2016). Maternal Factors are Important Predictors of Low Birth Weight: Evidence from Bangladesh Demographic & Health Survey-2011. *Malaysian Journal of Nutrition, 22*(2):257-265.

Rana M, Sayem A, Karim R, Islam N, Islam R, Zaman T K.(2015). Assessment of Knowledge regarding tuberculosis among non-medical university students in Bangladesh: A cross sectional study. *BMC Public Health*. 15:716. doi: 10.1186/s12889-015-2071-0.

Ravaoarisoa L, Randriamanantsaina L, Rakotonirina J, Marie JD, Donnen RP, Dramaix MW. (2018). Socioeconomic determinants of malnutrition among mothers in the Amoron'i Mania region of Madagascar: across-sectional study. *Nutrition* (2018) 4:6 https://doi. org/10.1186/s40795-018-0212-4.

Stevens GA, Finucane MM, De-Regil LM, Paciorek CJ, Flaxman SR, Branca F, PeñaRosas JP, Bhutta ZA, Ezzati M. (2013) Global, regional, and national trends in haemoglobin concentration and prevalence of total and severe anaemia in children and pregnant and non-pregnant women for 1995-2011: a systematic analysis of population-representative data. *Lancet Glob Health*. 2013 Jul;1(1):e16-25. doi: 10. 1016/S2214-109X(13)70001-9. Epub 2013 Jun 25.

Stevens, G. A., Finucane, M. M., Paciorek, C. J., Flaxman, S. R., White, R. A., Donner, A. J., Group, N. I. M. S. (2012). Trends in mild, moderate, and severe stunting and underweight, and progress towards MDG 1 in 141 developing countries: a systematic analysis of population representative data. *The Lancet*, 380(9844):824-834.

National Institute of Population Research and Training (NIPORT), Mitra and Associates, ICF International. Bangladesh Demographic and Health Survey, 2011. *NIPORT, Mitra & Associates and ICF International*, Dhaka, Bangladesh and Calverton, MD, USA. 2014.

National Institute of Population Research and Training (NIPORT), Mitra and Associates, ICF International. Bangladesh Demographic and Health Survey, 2011. *NIPORT, Mitra & Associates and ICF International*, Dhaka, Bangladesh and Calverton, MD, USA. 2013.

UNICEF (2017). *WHO, World Bank Group. Levels and Trends in Child Malnutrition in UNICEF/WHO/World Bank Group Joint Child Malnutrition Estimates Key Findings of the 2016 edition*. New York: UNICEF; Geneva: WHO; Washington DC: World Bank. Available at: http://www.who.int/nutgrowthdb/jme_brochoure.

Uddin, S. M., Hossain, M. G., Islam, M. A., Islam, M. N., Aik, S., &Kamarul, T. (2014). High-risk behavior of HIV/AIDS among females sex workers in Bangladesh: survey in Rajshahi City. *Japanese Journal of Infectious Diseases*, 67(3):191-196.

Victora, C. G., Adair, L., Fall, C., Hallal, P. C., Martorell, R., Richter, L., Group, C. U. S. (2008). Maternal and child under nutrition: consequences for adult health and human capital. *The Lancet*, 371(9609) :340-357.

World Health Organization. (2006). WHO child growth standards: length/height-for-age, weight-for-age, weight-for-length, weight-for-height and body mass index-for-age. *Methods and Development. WHO (non-serial publication). Geneva: WHO, 2007*. Available at: http:// www.who.int/childgrowth/standards/technical_report/en/.

WHO. 2017. *Fact sheet* http://www.who.int/topics/nutrition/en/.

In: Ethnicity and Syndrome X
Editors: M. Das and K. Bose

ISBN: 978-1-53618-042-8
© 2020 Nova Science Publishers, Inc.

Chapter 5

COMPARATIVE ANALYSIS OF TOTAL BODY PARAMETERS AND FUNCTIONAL CHARACTERISTICS OF MONGOLIAN RURAL AND URBAN CHILDREN AND ADOLESCENTS

Elena Z. Godina[1], L. Gundegmaa[2] and Ekaterina Yu. Permiakova[1]
[1] Anuchin Institute and Museum of Anthropology, Lomonosov Moscow State University, Moscow, Russia
[2]Mongolian National Institute of Physical Education, Ulaanbaatar, Mongolia

INTRODUCTION

Comparison of morphofunctional characteristics in urban and rural populations still remains one of the important goals in human biology. It is known that in the 18th and 19th centuries in some countries rural children were taller than their urban counterparts (Rona, 1984; Steegman, 1985; Bogin, 1988).

However, in the 20th century an opposite trend was revealed (Meredith, 1982; Eveleth, Tanner, 1990). Moreover, tempos of growth and development in urban children were much higher than in the rural ones (Miklashevskaya, Solovyeva, Godina, 1988; Wronska-Weclav, 1984). Urban children have bigger values of height and body weight but are lower in chest circumference (Wronska-Weclav, 1984; Chigea et al., 1987; Kozlov et al., 2008; Zhdanova, Starlukhova, Gurovich, 2014). They also have bigger values of Body Mass Index (BMI), which may be connected with less physical activity. Although recently it has been shown that physical load of children in rural areas is also going down (Permyakova, 2012; Liu et al., 2012). Comparison of modern urban and rural dwellers in Arkhangelsk region (Northern European part of Russian Federation) revealed that the urban children surpassed their rural counterparts in height but practically did not differ in the values of weight, chest circumference and BMI (Godina et al., 2017). Similar comparison of children in Arzamas area of Russia (Nizhny Novgorod region) revealed that rural children and adolescents of both sexes were characterized by higher values of weight but lower values of height than their urban peers (Kaluzhny, 2017). In subcutaneous fat layer evaluated as skinfold thickness rural children had lower values than the urban ones (Hajn, Komenda, 1985; Miklashevskaya, Solovyeva, Godina, 1988; Eveleth, Tanner, 1990; Gasser et al., 1993; Negasheva, 2008; Godina et al., 2011; Permyakova, 2012).

Analysis of recent trends in growth and development of rural and urban children in 141 countries allowed to conclude that urban children surpass their rural peers in mean values of height and weight but those trends were subjected to various secular changes in different regions. Thus, the differences were more expressed in the central and southern parts of South America, (Peru, Honduras, Bolivia and Guatemala); in some African states (Nigeria, Burundi, Burkina Faso); in Vietnam and China. In some other countries, like Chili and Brazil, this trend was much less expressed (Paciorek et al., 2013). Evaluation of morphological changes in Chinese children for the period from 1985 to 2014 revealed much higher values of height and weight in urban dwellers, the differences being more expressed in the samples examined in 1985-2000, with their further reduction. The authors explain these results with the impact of urbanization process (Ao et al., 2019).

As for Mongolia, the process of urbanization in this country has been rapidly increasing during the last 20 years. Thus, almost half of the Mongolian population now lives in the state capital - the city of Ulaanbaatar, although the living conditions are quite different: people can dwell in comfortable houses and apartments, or in the communal flats with shared facilities and even nomadic yurts[1], which exerts an influence on morphofunctional characteristics of children and adolescents (Gundegmaa, 2009).

Anthropological studies of peoples of Central Asia were carried out for the last 30 years, with significant contribution of the Russian researchers (Chikisheva, 1982; Antropoekologia Tsentral'noi Azii, 2005; Batsevich, Yasina, Sukhova, 2018). A special place in those studies was taken by Tatyana and Valery Alexeev who dedicated their research to the problem of interactions between humans and environment in different ecological zones of Central Asia including Mongolia (Antropoekologia Tsentral'noi Azii, 2005). However in recent years there were few studies dealing with differences in morphofunctional characteristics of urban and rural population of Mongolia. In the previous research it was shown that urban schoolchildren surpassed their rural peers in height, while in chest circumference the latter took the lead. However these differences were not statistically significant (Choibalsan, 1991).

Aim of the present paper is to characterize the patterns of growth processes in urban and rural Mongolian children in total body dimensions and some functional characteristics as well as to compare the results obtained in both groups.

---

[1] A traditional *yurt* (from the Turkic languages) or *ger* (Mongolian) is a portable, round tent covered with skins or felt and used as a dwelling by several distinct nomadic groups in the steppes of Central Asia.

Table 1. Numbers of investigated children by sex and age groups

Age, years	Boys		Girls	
	Urban	Rural	Urban	Rural
8	28	141	78	173
9	44	199	129	132
10	90	194	103	170
11	104	244	140	221
12	132	273	149	273
13	177	298	127	332
14	221	278	150	337
15	173	201	148	253
16	152	266	146	226
17	136	174	120	210
Total	1,257	2,268	1,290	2,327

Materials and Methods

The data for the present research were taken in 2013-2015 in the nation-wide study of 2,547 urban and 4,595 rural children and adolescents from 8 to 17 years old conducted in the central and southern regions of the country. The numbers of investigated children split by age and sex groups are given in Table 1.

The program of anthropometric investigation included the standard number of measurements (Bunak, 1941), of which only main/total measurements were used for the present analysis (height, weight, chest circumference), as well as Body Mass Index - BMI (Quetlet, 1871). Also the following functional characteristics were taken and analyzed - arterial blood pressure - systolic (SBP) and diastolic (DBP), heart rate (HR); grip strength of both hands. The material was collected cross-sectionally with the observance of bioethical procedure and signing of the informed concerned protocols. All data were depersonificated.

Statistical analysis was performed with the package “Statistica 8.0”. Main statistical parameters were calculated, significance of differences was evaluated with the Student’s t-test.

RESULTS

Comparison of Total Body Dimensions in Urban and Rural Children and Adolescents

Main statistical parameters of total body dimensions in different groups of Mongolian children and adolescents and the results of their comparison are given in Table 2.

Height

Analysis of age changes of this trait in boys of the two groups shows that up to the age of 13 years urban boys have higher mean values (the differences are statistically significant for the 8-12-year-olds ($p < 0.001$, - $p < 0.0001$)). At older ages the pattern changes, and at the age of 17 rural boys surpass their urban peers ($p < 0.001$). Significant differences in height between urban and rural girls are revealed at 9-10 and 12-13 years of age, urban girls being taller than their rural peers ($p < 0.001$). The increase in height stops in urban girls after the age of 13, and in the rural ones - after the age of 14. In the 17-year-olds the differences are not found (Table 2).

Weight

Analysis of age changes of weight in the two groups shows the presence of significant differences in 8-13-year-old boys and 11-17-year-old girls ($p < 0.001$, - $p < 0.0001$), directed towards bigger values of this parameter in urban dwellers (Table 2).

Body Mass Index

The trend towards bigger values of this parameter in those children who live in the city is preserved for the whole age range but statistically significant differences were observed only in 13- and 17-year-old boys ($p < 0.05$). For the girls the differences were statistically significant in 10-year-olds and at pubertal and post pubertal age groups (13-17 years).

Table 2. Descriptive characteristics of the total body dimensions of Mongolian urban and rural children and adolescents

Age, years	Height, cm				Weight, kg				BMI, kg/m^2				Chest circumference, cm			
	Urban		Rural		Urban		Rural		Urban		Rural		Urban		Rural	
	M	S	M	S	M	S	M	S	M	S	M	S	M	S	M	S
Boys																
8	127.6***	4.75	122.3***	7.87	26.4*	3.62	24.5*	4.80	16.2	1.66	16.3	2.37	59.5	2.75	58.2	3.23
9	133.5***	6.23	127.0***	6.13	30.1***	3.29	27.8***	3.99	16.8	1.83	17.2	2.07	60.7	3.19	60.0	3.50
10	138.7**	8.14	134.3***	6.27	33.7*	7.83	31.6*	6.52	17.3	2.57	17.5	2.74	64.5	4.39	64.3	4.70
11	143.4***	8.57	137.6***	6.50	37.3***	7.56	33.8***	6.39	18.0	2.97	17.8	2.55	66.4	6.81	66.2	4.96
12	149.0***	8.56	145.2***	8.60	42.1***	7.62	38.4***	6.88	18.8	2.57	18.2	2.37	70.2	6.50	70.0	5.18
13	153.2	8.64	153.0	8.75	46.2*	9.82	44.5*	7.68	19.5*	3.08	18.9*	2.27	70.2	7.80	70.0	6.28
14	156.6	9.89	158.0	9.83	49.0	9.22	49.0	8.47	19.8	2.73	19.5	2.38	76.7*	6.69	75.2*	6.20
15	162.1	9.68	162.2	8.44	52.2	9.37	52.3	8.77	19.9	3.66	19.8	2.35	79.2***	6.11	76.6***	6.14
16	165.3	7.58	166.3	7.86	56.7	7.12	56.5	8.53	20.7	2.04	20.4	2.16	80.9	8.04	81.1	6.28
17	167.2**	6.75	169.7**	6.52	62.2	8.26	60.8	7.43	22.2*	2.44	21.1*	2.17	85.0	5.05	85.1	7.01
Girls																
8	124.0	6.23	122.4	7.01	25.1	4.18	25.9	5.24	16.2**	1.73	17.2**	2.66	59.7***	3.86	54.8***	4.37
9	131.9**	7.53	128.5**	7.26	29.2	6.45	28.0	4.94	16.6	2.47	16.9	2.25	63.7***	6.14	59.6***	7.26
10	136.6	7.77	136.4	7.66	32.4	6.76	32.0	6.87	17.2*	2.10	16.4*	2.84	66.3***	5.21	61.7***	9.64
11	142.8	7.51	140.7	8.32	36.4**	7.91	34.7**	6.96	17.7	2.67	17.5	2.92	70.0***	3.61	66.8***	5.69
12	151.2**	8.11	148.0**	8.22	41.9***	7.27	39.6***	8.06	18.2	2.05	17.7	2.76	71.2	5.83	70.7	5.98
13	155.6**	6.52	151.9**	8.09	46.4***	7.35	42.5***	7.65	19.1**	2.36	18.3**	2.46	75.23*	7.04	73.9*	5.31
14	156.5	6.14	155.8	7.97	50.0***	7.90	46.3***	7.21	20.4***	2.82	19.1***	2.87	78.8***	4.43	75.6***	5.32
15	157.3	4.81	158.4	6.88	51.3**	7.74	49.5**	7.59	20.6**	2.88	19.7**	2.67	80.3***	5.57	77.8***	5.24
16	160.3	5.21	159.2	6.45	54.6***	6.78	51.2***	6.83	21.2**	2.35	20.2**	2.53	78.8	7.11	78.9	6.12
17	160.3	3.98	159.2	7.45	61.1***	4.02	53.6***	8.49	23.8***	1.15	21.1***	2.99	83.0***	4.68	80.6**	7.48

M = mean, S = standard deviation. Level of significance: $^{*}p < 0.05$, $^{**}p < 0.001$, $^{***}p < 0.0001$.

Chest Circumference

The results of the analysis show that significant differences for boys were revealed only at the age groups of 14-15 years when urban dwellers surpass their rural counterparts ($p < 0.05$ - $p < 0.001$), which could be due to the variations in biological age and tempos of growth in pubertal period. Urban girls surpass their rural peers practically at all age groups. Apart from 12- and 16-year-olds when the mean values of the above trait are identical in both groups studied (Table 2).

Comparison of Some Functional Characteristics in Urban and Rural Children and Adolescents

Main statistical parameters of some functional characteristics in different groups of Mongolian children and adolescents and the results of their comparison are given in Table 3.

Hand Grip Strength

The results of the analysis show (Table 3) that urban boys have lower values of right hand strength in 8-14 age groups when compared to the rural ones. These differences are statistically significant in 8-10- and 12-year-olds ($p < 0.05$ - $p < 0.001$). Starting from 14 years, the trend goes in the opposite direction, reaching the level of significance in 15-16-year-old youth ($p < 0.001$).

The results for the left hand strength are similar but changes in the vector occur earlier in life - after the age of 13 the urban dwellers surpass their rural peers in this characteristic (Table 3).

The same pattern was revealed for the girls: those who live in the city are stronger at all age groups, except for the period from 12 to 15 years, when no differences were found.

Table 3. Descriptive characteristics of the functional parameters of Mongolian urban and rural children and adolescents

Age	Right hand grip strength, kg				Left hand grip strength, kg				SBP, mm Hg.				DBP, mm Hg.				HR, b/min			
	Urban		Rural		Urban		Rural		Urban		Rural		Urban		Rural		Urban		Rural	
	M	S	M	S	M	S	M	S	M	S	M	S	M	S	M	S	M	S	M	S
Boys																				
8	21.2*	5.04	23.8*	5.25	18.9*	3.47	21.4*	4.95	109.7*	0.71	110.2	1.30	68.0*	2.93	69.3*	2.64	69.8**	2.70	71.2**	3.84
9	19.5***	10.53	24.2***	5.52	20.6*	11.37	23.4*	5.44	110.4**	2.83	112.1**	3.25	68.8**	2.38	70.5**	3.70	69.0**	2.85	70.1**	1.92
10	20.7*	12.44	23.2*	6.94	20.4	12.16	22.3	6.83	111.8**	3.33	113.3**	2.92	69.7***	1.93	72.1***	1.95	69.6**	2.32	70.7**	2.53
11	25.2	10.57	23.7	6.40	24.0*	9.70	21.9*	5.91	115.0	5.31	113.8	6.58	72.9***	5.42	75.0 ***	4.00	70.5***	2.35	72.2***	2.44
12	22.8***	8.88	26.4***	8.76	22.0**	9.43	24.5**	8.18	112.2**	4.31	116.4**	4.17	74.6	2.44	75.3	4.50	72.7	3.61	72.8	3.07
13	26.1	9.20	27.1	9.47	25.0	8.94	24.7	9.05	112.5**	4.23	117.1**	3.47	74.3***	2.49	75.8***	3.66	72.3*	2.34	73.0*	3.54
14	27.8	9.52	27.9	6.75	26.5	9.26	25.6	6.78	114.0**	4.58	116.5**	3.97	74.7	2.11	75.2	3.57	73.6**	2.08	72.7**	3.42
15	30.3***	8.60	27.0***	5.82	28.7**	8.44	25.8***	5.79	117.8**	5.51	115.1**	4.67	75.7*	4.64	74.4*	4.86	72.8	2.78	73.5	4.07
16	32.6***	11.30	28.8***	8.13	32.0***	11.90	27.2***	7.21	116.7	4.15	116.0	4.37	74.7	4.28	75.1	4.38	74.2*	4.80	73.4*	2.89
17	34.5	10.71	33.1	9.33	34.2*	11.05	31.4*	9.29	121.1**	5.14	116.5**	4.40	75.2	4.21	74.4	5.76	73.2**	4.61	75.0**	5.11
Girls																				
8	19.8***	6.49	11.2***	3.76	18.8***	6.29	9.9***	3.49	96.3	11.88	97.2	17.29	65.0	9.26	66.1	11.67	75.5	2.56	74.6***	7.94
9	17.4***	5.73	13.8***	5.83	16.3***	6.02	12.0***	4.59	91.8	7.80	97.2	12.68	62.3	7.14	62.3	9.22	76.9***	3.94	73.7***	6.12
10	20.6**	16.02	15.9**	7.96	19.8***	15.96	14.2***	7.78	94.4**	12.30	90.3**	9.16	66.1***	15.55	59.7***	8.82	78.4***	12.11	72.0***	7.21
11	18.7***	5.29	16.3***	4.98	17.4***	5.27	15.1***	4.34	92.7	6.64	90.9	12.66	63.3***	6.02	58.6***	10.19	77.6***	3.36	72.2***	6.82
12	19.4	5.63	19.7	6.43	18.4	5.25	18.1	5.58	91.6	6.02	90.9	12.07	62.7***	6.50	59.6***	10.04	77.3***	3.61	70.2***	6.07
13	20.4	6.09	20.5	5.09	19.9*	5.67	18.8*	4.79	98.7***	10.34	92.0***	12.42	69.2***	9.92	60.2***	10.08	74.2***	4.73	70.2***	6.42
14	22.1	14.22	22.0	5.69	21.3	13.91	20.0	4.96	99.6**	12.58	96.4**	10.32	71.1***	14.83	64.4***	8.58	75.4***	11.00	70.8***	5.29
15	23.8	9.65	22.9	6.32	22.3	8.49	21.4	5.83	101.1***	9.64	96.5***	9.95	70.6***	8.99	64.8***	7.30	73.8***	4.97	69.3***	5.54
16	25.7**	9.96	22.8**	8.08	24.3***	9.06	20.3***	6.06	103.4***	10.29	96.0***	9.84	70.0***	8.13	64.7***	7.46	73.7***	5.79	69.0***	5.91
17	27.4***	9.42	23.6***	6.38	26.3***	8.68	21.7***	5.47	104.2***	8.98	99.7***	11.32	73.6***	9.61	65.8***	8.55	74.6	6.62	73.7	9.22

M = mean, S = Standard Deviation. Level of significance: * $p < 0.05$, ** $p < 0.001$, *** $p < 0.0001$.

Arterial Blood Pressure and Heart Rate (SBP, DBP, HR).

Rural boys have bigger mean values of SBP up to 14 years of age (apart from 11-year-olds), after that age their urban peers prevail. Statistically significant differences were found at 8-10, 12-15 and 17 years of age). The same trend is typical for DBP: larger values of this trait occur in the rural schoolchildren at the age of 8-14 years, with the further changes in the opposite direction. The differences are significant in 8-11- and 13-year-olds (Table 3).

In girls, the SBP values are bigger in those who live in the city, starting from the age of 10 years (at 10, 13-17 years of age the differences are significant). DBP mean values are higher in the urban girls practically at all ages starting from 9 years, with high level of significance (Table 3).

For HR values the differences are almost the same. In boys the rural dwellers have bigger values at some age groups (8-11, 13- and 17-year-olds), while in 14- and 16-year-olds an opposite direction of differences is found. In girls at all ages the HR means are higher for the capital inhabitants (Table 3).

DISCUSSION

The differences in height between urban and rural Mongolian children and adolescents may serve as an indicator of changes in the socioeconomic conditions in the country. Thus, in the middle of the last century no such differences were found, or, if found, did not reach the level of statistical significance (Chultemdorzh, 1967).

It was shown early that for the period from 1975 to 2010 height and weight of Mongolian children significantly increased due to the rapid socioeconomic transformations (Gundegmaa, 2009; Godina et al., 2019). However, deficit of weight and short stature are still found in some poor rural areas due to existing inequality in food resources and the level of socioeconomic development (Altantsetseg, 2015; Paciorek et al., 2013). Urban Mongolian children of both sexes have higher values in weight than their rural peers, practically at all age groups, except for 14-16-year-old boys. It should be emphasized that in girls this trend is more clearly expressed. Previously it was found that for the period from 1975 to 2010, height and weight of Mongolian children significantly increased due to socioeconomic transformations taken place in the country (Paciorek et al., 2013). Our results seem quite logical in this context.

The differences in BMI are also mostly expressed in case of the girls: urban inhabitants have bigger values of this parameter, particularly at older age groups. It is mainly connected with bigger values of weight in the former, due to better quality of food and life in the city and especially in the capital of the country. These results confirm previously published data by other researchers (Amgalan, Pogorelova, 2015; Pogorelova, Amgalan, 2016).

The means of chest circumference are bigger in the urban dwellers of both sexes when compared to the rural ones, the differences, again, being more expressed in the girls (Table 3). This result does not coincide with the conclusion of the study made by Choibolsan that rural children surpassed their urban peers in this parameter (Choibalsan, 1991). However, our results are similar to some other studies, which showed larger values of chest circumference in urban children, particularly at older ages (Reztsova, 1995; Permyakova, 2012).

It should be noted that in the classical anthropological literature the values of chest circumference were always bigger in the inhabitants of villages, which was considered as one of the typical characteristics of their body structure (Bashkirov, 1962).

The results for functional characteristics show that in the grip strength of both hands urban boys are weaker than their rural peers up to the age of 13 but surpass them after that age. This could be explained by the differences in the life style of rural and urban dwellers, the former being involved in significant physical activity starting from early age. They help their parents with agricultural works, household loads, etc. However, the city dwellers have more access to various kinds of physical training: sports schools, section and clubs. Urban children, particularly at older ages, are very much interested in their physical appearance, influenced by mass media stereotypes, and start actively doing some physical exercises or going in for sport. That is why they finally surpass their rural peers in strength indicators.

As for the girls, those living in the city are stronger than their rural peers during all of the studied period. Rural girls are much weaker than their urban counterparts at all ages. These results do not support, however, the conclusions received early by Altantsetseg (2015) for the northern regions of Mongolia, where rural children surpass their urban peers in physical strength. This contradiction could be explained by the differences in the city samples: for the present study the children of Mongolian capital were investigated, while in the previous case urban children were represented by the dwellers of much smaller towns.

As in the case of chest circumference, it should be noted again that in the classical anthropological studies physical fitness of rural population was always considered as one of its basic characteristics (Bashkirov, 1962). But living conditions are changing and as a result in many populations nowadays rural dwellers are becoming physically weaker than their urban peers.

When some hemodynamic characteristics were compared, it turned out that urban boys up to the age 14 had lower values of BP and HR, while later in life they surpass their rural peers in these indicators. In girls, urban dwellers had much higher values of blood pressure and HR at all age groups. It could be considered as an indicator of unfavorable stress impact on those living in the big city (Negasheva et al., 2018).

It is also worth noting that for most of the studied traits, clearly expressed gender differences were found. In girls more statistically significant differences were found and the level of statistical significance was also higher. The same trends were revealed in the study of secular changes in Mongolian children and adolescents (Godina et al., 2019). It may be also concluded that in this case, like in many others, the direction of spatial and temporal changes are parallel.

Conclusion

The revealed differences in the values of morphofunctional indicators of urban and rural children suggest the continuing impact of urbanization on the physical condition in the surveyed groups. Urban children have larger values of total body dimensions and surpass their rural counterparts in physical strength, which could be explained by their having access to some special programs of physical training. Changes in hemodynamic parameters in the direction of their increase in the city dwellers are likely to be associated with excessive stress load in urban environments.

Acknowledgments

This work was supported by the research project № AAAA-A19-119013090163-2 "Anthropology of Eurasian populations" and partly by Moscow State University Grant for Leading Scientific Schools "Depository of the Living Systems" in frame of the MSU Development Program.

References

Altantsetseg L. Pedagogicheskie osnovy diversifikacii regional'nyh programm po fizicheskomu vospitaniyu na osnove sravnitel'nogo analiza rezul'tatov morfofunkcional'nogo razvitiya i fizicheskoj podgotovlennosti shko'nikov razlichnyh ajmakov Mongolii [Pedagogical bases of diversification of regional programs in physical education based on a comparative analysis of the results of morphofunctional development and physical fitness of schoolchildren of various aimags of Mongolia]. *Avtoref. diss. ... dokt. ped. nauk* [*Abstract of dissertation ... Doc. of. Sc. in pedagogy*], Moscow, 2015. 297 p. (In Russ.).

Amgalan G., Pogorelova I. G. Analiz pokazatelej fizicheskogo razvitiya 7-16-letnih shkol'nikov Mongolii [Analysis of indicators of physical development of 7-16-year-old schoolchildren of Mongolia], *Sibirskij medicinskij zhurnal* [*Siberian Medical Journal*], 2015, 1, pp. 88-90. (In Russ.).

Antropoekologiya Tsentral'noj Azii. Otv. red. T. I. Alekseeva, V. A. Bacevich, R. M. Munchaev, O. M. Pavlovskii, B. B. Prohorov, V. A. Spitsin [*Anthropoecology of Central Asia*. Eds. T. I. Alekseeva, V. A. Batsevich, R. M. Munchaev, O. M. Pavlovsky, B. B. Prokhorov, V. A. Spizyn], Moscow, Nauchnyj mir Publ., 2005, pp. 6-126. (In Russ.).

Ao D., Wu F., Yun C. F., Zheng X. Y. Trends in Physical Fitness Among 12-Year-Old Children in Urban and Rural Areas During the Social Transformation Period in China. *J. Adolesc. Health*, 2019, 64 (2), pp. 250-257. doi: 10.1016/j.jadohealth.2018.08.021.

Bashkirov P. N. *Uchenie o fizicheskom razvitii cheloveka*. [*The Study of Human Physical Development*]. Moscow, Moscow State University Publ., 1962. 339 p. (In Russ.)

Batsevich V. A., Yasina O. V., Sukhova A. V. Secular and Age-Related Dynamics of Biological Characteristics in the Rural Population of Mongolia: A Study of Environmental Adaptation. *Archaeology, Ethnology & Anthropology of Eurasia*, 2018, 46 (1), pp. 144-153. doi: 10.17746/1563-0110.2018.46.1.

Bogin B. A. *Rural-to-urban migration, Biological Aspects of Human Migration*, Ed. C. G. N. Mascie-Taylor. Cambridge: Cambridge Univ. Press, 1988. P. 90-129.

Bunak V. V. *Antropometriya* [*Anthropometry*]. Moscow, Uchpedgiz Publ., 1941. 368 p. (In Russ.).

Chigea S., Miu G., Tudoscie A. Variabiletatea ecologica a tipulue constitucional intervalul de virsta 17-20 de ani. *Stud. si cerc* [The ecological variability of the constitutional type has the age range of 17-20 years]. *Antropol.*, 1987, 24, pp. 48-55.

Chikisheva, T. A. Izuchenie svyazi antropologicheskih osobennostej naseleniya s ekologicheskimi faktorami (na primere Altae-Sayanskogo regiona) [Studying the relationship of anthropological features of the population with environmental factors (for example, the Altai-Sayan region)]. *Avtoref. diss. ...kand. biol. nauk* [*Abstract of dissertation ... Ph. D. in biology*], Moscow, 1982, 23 p. (In Russ.).

Choibalsan L. Normativnye trebovaniya k fizicheskomu razvitiyu i fizicheskoj podgotovlennosti doprizyvnoj molodezhi (16-18 let) MNR [Regulatory requirements for the physical development and physical fitness of pre-conscription youth (16-18 years old) of the MNR]. *Avtoref. diss. ...kand. biol. nauk* [*Abstract of dissertation ... Ph. D. in pedagogy*], M., 1991, 28 p. (In Russ.).

Chultemdorzh Ch. Suragchdyn bie byaldryn hugzhiltyin zarim asuudald, Ulsyn hevleliyn hereg erhleh gazar. Ulan-Bator, 1967. 51 x. (In Mongol.).

Eveleth P. B., Tanner J. M. *Worldwide variation and human growth*. 2nd ed., P. B. Eveleth, J. M. Tanner. Cambridge University Press, 1990. 268 p.

Gasser, R. B., Chilton, N. B., Hoste, H. Beveridge, I. Rapid sequencing of rDNA from single worms and eggs of parasitic helminths. *Nucleic Acids Res.*, 1993, 21, pp. 2525-2526.

Godina E. Z., Khomyakova I. A., Zadorozhnaya L. V. Patterns of Growth and Development in Urban and Rural Children of the Northern Part of European Russia. *Archaeology, Ethnology and Anthropology of Eurasia,* 2017, 45 (1), pp. 146-156. doi: 10.17746/1563-0102.2017.45.1.

Godina E. Z., Khomyakova I. A., Zadorozhnaya L. V., Anisimova A. V., Ivanova E. M., Permyakova E. Yu., Svistunova N. V., Stepanova A. V., Gilyarova O. A., Zubareva V. V. Auksologicheskie issledovaniya na rodine M. V. Lomonosova [Auxological studies at the homeland of M. V. Lomonosov]. *Vestnik Moskovskogo universiteta. Seriya XXIII. Antropologiya* [*Moscow University Anthropology Bulletin*], 2011, 3, pp. 68-100. (In Russ.).

Godina Elena Z., Lhagvasuren Gundegmaa, Shagdar Bat-Erdene, Zadorozhnaya Liudmila V., Permiakova Ekaterina Yu, Khomiakova Irina A. Secular Changes in Mongolia: Shift in Tempos of Growth. *Collegium Antropologicum*, 2019, 43, № 1, 11-20.

Gundegmaa L. Morphofunktsional'nye osobennosti studencheskoi molodezhi Mongolii v zavisimosti ot sredovykh I geneticheskykh factorov [Morphofunctional Characteristics of Mongolian youth under the influence of environmental and genetic factors*]. Diss... kand. biol. Nauk, M.*, 2009, (In Russ.).

Hajn V., Komenda S. Zur Menarche - Problematic der Madchen und ihrer Mutter aus Olomouc. *Anthropologie* (CSSR), 1985, 23 (1), pp. 5-19.

Kalyuzhnyj E. A. Auksologicheskie aspekty antropometricheskih skriningov uchashchihsya goroda i rajona Nizhegorodskoj oblasti [Auxological aspects of anthropometrical screenings of urban and rural students of Nizhny Novgorod Region]. Vestnik Moskovskogo universiteta. Seriya XXIII. *Antropologiya* [*Moscow University Anthropology Bulletin*], 2017, 3, pp. 86-93. (In Russ.).

Kozlov A. I., Vershubskaya G. G., Popovskij A. I., Sanina E. D. Fizicheskoe razvitie gorodskih i sel'skih shkol'nikov Gornomarijskogo rajona Respubliki Marij-El [Physical development of urban and rural schoolchildren of Gornomariysky district of the Republic of Mari El]. *Novye issledovaniya* [*New research*], 2008, 2, pp. 14-21. (In Russ.).

Liu J. H., Jones S. J., Sun H., Probst J. C., Merchant A. T., Cavicchia P. Diet, physical activity, and sedentary behaviors as risk factors for childhood obesity: an urban and rural comparison. *Child. Obes.*, 2012, 8 (5), pp. 440-448.

Meredith, P., Dengate, H. N., Morrison, W. R. The Lipids of Various Sizes of Wheat Starch Granules. *Starch*, 1978, 30 (4), pp. 119-125.

Miklashevskaya N. N., V. S. Solov'eva, E. Z. Godina. Rost i razvitie abkhazskich detey i podrostkov [Growth and development of the Abkhazian children and adolescents]. In: *Rostovye prozessy u detey i podrostkov* [*Growth Processes in Children and Adolescents*]. Moscow, MSU Publ., 1988, pp. 112-144. (In Russ.).

Negasheva M. A. Morfologicheskaya konstituciya cheloveka v yunosheskom periode ontogeneza (integral'nye aspekty) [The morphological constitution of a person in the youthful period of ontogenesis (integral aspects)]. *Avtoref. diss. ... dokt. ped. nauk*

[*Abstract of dissertation ... Doc. of. Sc. in biology*], Moscow, 48 p. (In Russ.).

Negasheva M. A., Zimina S. N., Sineva I. M., Yudina A. M. Osobennosti morfofunkcional'noj adaptacii studencheskoj molodezhi, prozhivayushchej v raznyh gorodah Rossii [Characteristic features of morphofunctional adaptation of young students living in different cities of Russia]. Vestnik Moskovskogo universiteta. Seriya 23: *Antropologiya* [*Moscow University Anthropology Bulletin*], 2018, 3, pp. 41-54. (In Russ.).

Paciorek C. J., Stevens G. A., Finucane M. M., Ezzati M. Nutrition Impact Model Study Group (Child Growth). Children's height and weight in rural and urban populations in low-income and middle-income countries: a systematic analysis of population-representative data. *Lancet. Glob. Health*, 2013, 1 (5), pp. 300-309.

Permyakova, E. Yu. Sovremennye tendencii razvitiya zhirootlozheniya ugorodskih i sel'skih detej i podrostkov [Current trends in the development of fat deposition in urban and rural children and adolescents]. *Avtoref. diss. ...kand. biol. nauk* [*Abstract of dissertation ... Ph. D. in biology*], Moscow, 2012, 26 p. (In Russ.).

Pogorelova I. G., Amgalan G. Kharakteristika fizicheskogo razvitiya shkol'nikov Mongolii i faktorov, ego formiruyushchih [Characteristics of the physical development of schoolchildren of Mongolia and the factors shaping it]. *Gigiena i sanitariya* [*Hygiene and sanitation*], 2016, 95. (12), pp. 1198-1201. (In Russ.).

Quetlet A. Antropometrie, A. Quetlet. *Bruxelas*, 1871. 251 p.

Reztsova E. M. Sravnitel'naya kharakteristika fizicheskogo i biologicheskogo razvitiya detej shkol'nogo vozrasta, prozhivayushchih v g. Kirove i sel'skoj mestnosti Kirovskoj oblasti Rossijskoj Federacii [Comparative characteristics of the physical and biological development of school-age children living in the city of Kirov and the countryside of the Kirov region of the Russian Federation]. *Avtoref. diss. ... dokt. ped. nauk* [*Abstract of dissertation ... Kand. Sc. in medicine*], 1995, 18 p. (In Russ.).

Rona R. J. Ecological environment, In: *Genetic and Environmental factors during Growth Period.* Ed. C. Susanne. N. Y., London: Plenum Press, 1984, pp. 199-207.

Steegman A. T. (Jr.) 18th century British military stature: growth cessation, selective recruiting, secular trends, nutrition at birth, cold and occupation. *Hum. Biol.*, 1985, 57 (1), pp. 775-795.

Wronska-Weclaw W. Dynamics of growth and maturation of countryside children in selected region of Poland. *Stud. Hum. Ecol.*, 1984, 5, pp. 241-272.

Zhdanova O. A., Stahurlova L. I., Gurovich O. V. Sravnitel'naya ocenka fizicheskogo razvitiya shkol'nikov, prozhivayushchih v gorodskih i sel'skih poseleniya Voronezhskoj oblasti [Comparative assessment of the physical development of schoolchildren living in urban and rural settlements of the Voronezh region]. *Nauchno-medicinskij vestnik Central'nogo Chernozem'ya* [*Scientific Medical Herald of the Central Black Soil Region*], 2014, 57, pp. 24-28. (In Russ.).

In: Ethnicity and Syndrome X
Editors: M. Das and K. Bose
ISBN: 978-1-53618-042-8
© 2020 Nova Science Publishers, Inc.

Chapter 6

METABOLIC SYNDROME AMONG INDIAN FEMALES: A REVIEW

Ramanpreet Randhawa**[*] **and Sharda Sidhu
Department of Human Genetics, Guru Nanak Dev University,
Amritsar, Punjab, India

INTRODUCTION

Metabolic Syndrome (MS) or syndrome X is a major, widely prevalent and escalating public health challenge in both developed and developing countries (Ford, 2004; Grundy, 2008; Xi et al., 2013; Hajian-Tilaki, 2015; Owolabi et al., 2017). It has been described as a global time bomb, with a quarter of the world's adult population estimated to be having this condition and many more are prone to it (Awosan et al., 2013; Jain et al., 2015). The metabolic syndrome consists of a constellation of metabolic abnormalities like obesity, hypertension, T2DM and dyslipidemia. It is emerging as one of the major public health problem tend to aggregate metabolic abnormalities

[*]Corresponding Author's Email: raman.randhawa19@gmail.com.

in individuals and that clustering is more harmful than having a single metabolic component in an individual (Kimm et al.,2004; Mohammadbeigi et al.,2011). It has gained attention, because it makes an individual vulnerable to various Cardiovascular Diseases (CVDs), including Coronary Artery Disease (CAD), various cerebrovascular and peripheral vascular diseases necessitating long-term health care, Polycystic Ovarian Syndrome (PCOS), musculo-skletal disorders, fatty liver, gall bladder disease, kidney disease, eye disorders, hormonal imbalances, asthma, sleep apnea and certain forms of cancer (Isomaa et al., 2001; Zimmet et al., 2005; Alberti et al., 2006,2009). Individuals with metabolic syndrome have two-fold risk of developing CVDs, three-fold risk of heart attack and five-fold risk of developing Type 2 Diabetes Mellitus (T2DM) than without metabolic syndrome subjects (Cornier et al., 2008; Sawant et al., 2011). It was also reported by Alberti et al. (2009) that among individuals after diagnosis of metabolic syndrome, the risk of developing CVD increases over the next five to ten years.CVD is one of the leading causes of death among women in the world (Lloyd-Jones et al., 2009). It is estimated that half of all cardiovascular events in women are related to MS (Carr, 2003). The studies have indicated that women aged more than 55 have a higher incidence of CVD than younger women (Lerner and Kannel, 1986; Ford et al., 2002; Rosamund et al., 2007). It was demonstrated by Lakka et al. (2002) that metabolic syndrome is a high risk condition for overall cardiovascular mortality. This relationship was first documented in middle-aged adults but nowadays this association exists at an early age accounting in part for early CVD. It is now well known that metabolic syndrome is an acknowledged predictor for all-cause morbidity and mortality across the globe (Zimmet et al., 2005; Alberti et al., 2006).

The epidemiological significance of MS as a tool for identifying individuals at high risk of cardiovascular diseases is essential to estimate the prevalence of metabolic syndrome at population levels because metabolic syndrome poses a huge financial and psychological burden on the individuals and societies. The purpose of this review article was to assemble information about the prevalence of MS from different regions of India, as accurate estimates of prevalence of MS are necessary to plan effective control measures.

Materials and Methods

A study protocol, search strategies and study eligibility criteria were prepared. The medical search engines, namely PubMed/Medline (National Library of Medicine, Bethesda, MD, USA) Research Gate, NCBI, Embase, Cochrane Library, Academic Search, Web of Science, Scopus, Google Scholar, JSTOR, Science Direct and Govt. Websites of South Asians, were used for literature search using multiple keywords, "Metabolic Syndrome (MS), background of MS, diagnosis of MS, diagnostic criteria of MS, prevalence of MS in Indian females, association of MS with menstrual status, MS and cardiovascular diseases, urban and rural Indian females studies on MS." A manual search was also made using cross-references mentioned in various research papers, and a contact was established with various researchers and scientists for further information. The search was restricted to the studies published from the year 2003 to 2019. For the present review article, 50 epidemiological studies were identified of which 6 were excluded based on the inclusion criteria and 44 were considered for data extraction. The eligibility criteria for inclusion in this review article were (i) Metabolic Syndrome was assessed using any of these five internationally recognised and valid criteria named as World Health Organization (WHO, 1999), National Cholesterol Education Program Adult Treatment Panel-III (NCEP ATP-III, 2001), International Diabetes Federation (IDF, 2005), modified NCEP ATP-III (mNCEP ATP-III, 2005), and Joint Interim Statement (JIS, 2009) also known as Harmonized Asian-Specific Diagnostic Criterion. Details of these criteria are given below in Table 1. (ii) Population based epidemiological studies in which the prevalence of metabolic syndrome among Indian females was reported and (iii) studies conducted among adult Indian females (age $\geq$17 years). On the other hand, 8 studies which did not satisfy the inclusion criteria were excluded like male-oriented studies, paediatric studies, case-control studies and cohort studies.

Table 1. Five internationally renowned diagnostic criteria of metabolic syndrome

Diagnostic Criteria	Components of Metabolic Syndrome (MS)							Assessment of Metabolic Syndrome
	Obesity			T2DM	Hypertension	Dyslipidemia		
	BMI (kg/m²)	WHR	WC (cm)	FBG (mg/dl)	BP (mmHg)	TGL (mg/dl)	HDL-C (mg/dl)	
WHO (1999)	≥ 30	> 0.85	-----	≥110	≥140/90	≥150	<39	Glucose intolerance plus any two risk factors
NCEP ATP-III (2001)	-----	-----	≥ 88	≥110	≥130/85	≥150	≤50	At least any three risk factors
IDF (2005)	-----	-----	≥ 80	≥100	≥130/85	≥150	≤50	Abdominal obesity plus any two risk factors
mNCEP ATP-III (2005)	-----	-----	≥ 80	≥110	≥130/85	≥150	≤50	At least any three risk factors
JIS (2009)	-----	-----	≥ 80	≥100	≥130/85	≥150	≤50	At least any three risk factors

International Diabetes Federation (IDF).
Joint Interim Statement (JIS).
Modified National Cholesterol Education Program Adult Treatment Panel- III (mNCEP ATP-III).
National Cholesterol Education Program Adult Treatment Panel- III (NCEP ATP-III).
World Health Organization (WHO).

RESULTS

The prevalence of MS among adult Indian females in various regions of India evaluated on the basis of five internationally recognized diagnostic criteria, namely WHO (1999), NCEP ATP-III (2001), IDF (2005), mNCEPATP-III (2005), and JIS (2009) is summarized in Table 2.

Table 2. Percentage prevalence of Metabolic Syndrome (MS) among adult females reported in various Indian studies

Place/Area/State	Age group (years)	No. of females	Percentage prevalence of MS using different diagnostic criteria					Investigator
			WHO (1999)	NCEP ATP-III (2001)	NCEP mATP-III (2005)	IDF (2005)	JIS (2009)	
Northern Region								
Amritsar/Punjab	40-65	1520	13.1	41.5	46.4	47.5	52.1	Randhawa and Sidhu (2019)
Udhampur/Jammu & Kashmir	≥18	101	---	51.3	---	53.9	---	Sharma et al. (2019)
Uttar Pradesh	≥30	188	---	59.0	---	---	---	Khan et al. (2018)
Uttar Pradesh	≥18	---	---	20.3	---	---	---	Bansal et al. (2017)
Uttar Pradesh	≥18	-	---	---	13.8	---	---	Zafar et al. (2017)
Haryana	---	882	---	---	---	38.2	---	Singh et al. (2016)
Sultanpur Lodhi/ Kapurthala/Punjab	≥20	177	---	---	57.3	---	---	Kaur (2014)
Ambala/ Haryana	≥20	627	---	---	---	11.6	---	Pathania et al. (2013)
Delhi	35-65	413	---	---	55.1	---	---	Sharma and Mahna (2012)
Srinagar	---	243	---	9.9	---	---	---	Bhat et al. (2010)
Chandigarh	≥18	315	---	44.8	---	---	59.6	Mangat et al. (2010)
Southern Region								
Kochi//Kerala	20-60	183	---	67.8	---	---	---	Vatakencherry and Saraswathy (2019)
Tamil Nadu	≥20	302	---	---	66.2	65.9	---	Meenakshi et al. (2019)
Karnataka	17-23	67	---	---	---	11.9	---	Teli et al. (2019)
Kerala	20-79	3035	---	35.2	---	39.5	---	Harikrishnan et al. (2018)
Hyderabad//Telangana	18-75	110	---	---	---	58.1	---	Allam et al. (2018)

Table 2. (Continued)

Place/Area/State	Age group (years)	No. of females	Percentage prevalence of MS using different diagnostic criteria					Investigator
			WHO (1999)	NCEP ATP-III (2001)	NCEP mATP-III (2005)	IDF (2005)	JIS (2009)	
Northern Region								
Karnataka	---	---	---	35.8	---	---	---	Sarkar et al. (2016)
Khozikode/ Kerala	≥20	327	---	---	28.1	---	---	Roshni et al. (2014)
Chennai	33-59	---	---	42.2	---	---	---	Padmavathi et al. (2013)
Tumpur/ Karnataka	≥18	590	---	---	57.9	---	---	Shalini et al. (2013)
Tumpur/ Karnataka	≥18	433	---	---	55.1	---	---	Shalini et al. (2013)
Karnataka	≥20	500	---	---	---	31.2	---	Pemminati et al. (2010)
Chennai	≥20	1254	19.7	19.4	---	28.2	---	Deepa et al. (2007)
Madras/ Tamil Nadu	20-75	217	---	---	46.5	---	---	Ramachandran et al. (2003)
Western Region								
Surendranagar/ Gujarat	20-80	---	---	---	---	---	44.2	Chinawale et al. (2018)
Ahmedabad/ Gujarat	25-65	265	---	34.6	---	54.8	---	Patel et al. (2016)
Mumbai/ Maharashtra	18-26	176	---	22.0	---	7.0	---	Jadhavet al. (2014)
Mandur/ Goa	≥20	176	---	---	39.8	---	---	Peixoto and Shah et al. (2014)
Mumbai/ Maharashtra	20-90	246	---	---	12.6	---	---	Sawant et al. (2011)
Mumbai/ Maharashtra	35-66	498	---	---	---	56.6	58.4	Pandey et al. (2010)
Wardha/ Mumbai/ Maharashtra	≥18	131	---	7.6	---	---	---	Kamble et al. (2010)
Jaipur/ Rajasthan	≥20	840	---	39.9	---	---	---	Gupta et al. (2004)
Eastern Region								
Kolkatta/West Bengal	18-49	---	---	---	---	55.6	---	Banerjee et al. (2019)

Place/Area/State	Age group (years)	No. of females	Percentage prevalence of MS using different diagnostic criteria					Investigator
			WHO (1999)	NCEP ATP-III (2001)	NCEP mATP-III (2005)	IDF (2005)	JIS (2009)	
Place/Area/State	Age group (years)	No. of females	Percentage prevalence of MS using different diagnostic criteria					Investigator
			WHO (1999)	NCEP ATP-III (2001)	NCEP mATP-III (2005)	IDF (2005)	JIS (2009)	
Odisha	≤40	53	---	---	28.3	---	---	Manjareeka et al. (2018)
Dibrugarh/Assam	20-60	---	---	---	51.1	---	---	Mahanta et al. (2017)
Kolkatta/ West Bengal	18-24	235	---	---	---	---	6.0	Das et al. (2017)
West Bengal	45-70	222	---	---	---	45.9	---	Srimani et al. (2017)
Imphal/ Manipur	21-70	237	---	21.0	---	---	---	Rothangpui et al. (2015)
Dibrugarh/ Assam	≥20	233	---	---	---	45.9	---	Kotokey et al. (2013)
Behrampur/ Orissa	20-80	307	---	---	---	---	52.2	Prasad et al. (2012)
West Bengal	≥18	128	---	48.4	---	---	---	Sarkar et al. (2006)
Tribal females/ West Bengal(Toto and Bhutia)	≥18	150 46	---	3.8 52.2	---	---	---	Sarkar et al. (2006)
Central Region								
Indore/ Madhya Pradesh	20-80	259	---	---	8.1	---	---	Agrawal et al. (2017)
Town in Central India	≥20	267	---	13.5	---	---	---	Jain et al. (2015)

For studying the prevalence rates of MS in India all the collected studies were categorised into five groups (Northern, Southern, Western, Eastern and Central Region) on the basis of regional background where the studies were conducted. Out of 44 epidemiological studies, 11 from Northern Region, 13 from Southern Region, 08 from Western Region, 10 from Eastern Region and 02 from Central Region were included. The number of participants in all these studies ranged from 53 to 3035.Among adult females of India, the prevalence rate of MS varied from 9.9%-59.6% in Northern Region, 11.9%-67.8% in Southern Region, 7.6%-58.4% in Western Region and 3.8%-55.6% in Eastern Region. Overall, the highest prevalence of MS [67.8%; NCEP ATP-III (2001)] was observed in Kerala state of Southern region by Vatakencherry and Saraswathy (2019) and the lowest prevalence [3.8%; NCEP ATP-III (2001)] among Toto tribal females in West Bengal state of sub-Himalayan region assessed by Sarkar et al. (2006).

In Northern Region studies, the maximum prevalence of MS (59.6%, JIS)was observed in the women of Chandigarh depicted by Mangat et al. (2010) followed by population of Uttar Pradesh (59.0%; NCEP ATP-III), Punjab; the prevalence of metabolic syndrome was 57.3% in females of Sultanpur lodhi, Kapurthala according to mNCEP ATP-III criterion (Kaur, 2014), Delhi (55.1%; mNCEP ATP-III) estimated by Sharma and Mahna (2012), Jammu and Kashmir 101 females aged ≥18 years were screened with 53.9% estimates of MS using IDF guidelines (Sharma et al., 2019), 52.1% prevalence of MS was detected on the basis ofJIS criterion among 1520 women ranging in age 40-60 years of Amritsar district of Punjab (Randhawa and Sidhu, 2019), Jammu and Kashmir (51.3%; NCEP ATP-III), 47.5% and 46.4% estimates of MS on applying IDF and mNCEP ATP-III guidelines were found among women of Amritsar district of Punjab by Randhawa and Sidhu (2019), Chandigarh (44.8%, NCEP ATP-III) diagnosed by Mangat et al. (2010), Punjab;41.5% according to NCEP ATP-III among females of Amritsar diagnosed by Randhawa and Sidhu (2019), 38.2% prevalence of MS was estimated by Singh et al. (2016) among 882 women of Haryana as per IDF standard, 20.3% (NCEP ATP-III) and 13.8% (mNCEP ATP-III) women of Uttar Pradesh were investigated by Bansal et al. (2017) and Zafar et al. (2017), respectively, Amritsar district of Punjab (13.1%, WHO) revealed by Randhawa and Sidhu (2019), 627 women of Haryana demonstrated 11.6% prevalence of MS according to IDF method studied by Pathania et al. (2013) and the least prevalence of metabolic syndrome in Northern region was 9.9% (NCEP ATP-III criterion) depicted by females of Srinagar according to Bhat et al. (2010).

In Southern region studies, 67.8% was recognised as the highest prevalence of MS using NCEP ATP-III guidelines among Kerala females by Vatakencherry and Saraswathy (2019) followed by women of Tamil Nadu (mNCEP ATP-III: 66.2%; IDF: 65.9%) investigated by Meenakshi et al. (2019). An investigation performed by Allam et al. (2018) among Telangana women postulated 58.1% estimates of metabolic syndrome on the basis of IDF method. In Karnataka (57.9%, mNCEP ATP-III) revealed through a study done on 590 females by Shalini et al. (2013). In the same region, Shalini et al.(2013) studied 433 females aged 18 years and above residing in Tumpur district of Karnataka and reported 55.1% prevalence of metabolic syndrome as per mNCEP ATP-III standard. In Tamil Nadu 2003, Ramachandran et al., found 46.5% prevalence of metabolic syndrome among Tamil Nadu females as per mNCEP ATP-III diagnostic criterion, Chennai; a study conducted on Chennai females (aged 33-59 years) by Padmavathi et al. (2013) reported 42.2% prevalence of metabolic syndrome when NCEP ATP-III standard was applied, Kerala (39.5%, IDF) reported by Harikrishnan et al. (2018), Karnataka;Sarkar et al.(2016) observed the metabolic syndrome prevalence as 35.8% using NCEP ATP-III guidelines, Kerala (35.2%, NCEP ATP-III) among 3035 women screened by Harikrishnan et al. (2018), Karnataka; the study carried out by Pemminati et al. (2010) observed 31.2% Karnataka females suffering with metabolic syndrome on the basis of IDF definition.Chennai; Deepa et al. (2007) employed dianostic criteria i.e., IDF to assess the prevalence of metabolic syndrome among Chennai females and observed 28.2% females were falling in the category of MS, Kerala; in another study, among Kerala women (≥20 years) the prevalence of metabolic syndrome was observed as 28.1% as per mNCEP ATP-III criterion by Roshni et al. (2014), Chennai; Deepa et al. (2007) employed two diagnostic criteria i.e., WHO and NCEP ATP-III to determine the estimates of metabolic syndrome among Chennai females and revealed 19.7% and 19.4% females suffering with MS and the lowest(11.9%) prevalence of metabolic syndrome was diagnosed among Karnataka females using IDF criterion by Teli et al. (2019).

In Western Region studies, the maximum prevalence of MS (JIS: 58.4%; IDF: 56.6)was observed in the women of Maharashtra determined by Pandey et al. (2010), Gujarat in another study, among Gujarati women aged 25-65 years the prevalence of metabolic syndrome was 54.8% on employing IDF guidelines (Patel et al. 2016), Gujarat; 44.2% women were observed in the category of metabolic syndrome using JIS (2009) guidelines by Chinawale et al. (2018), 39.9% of Gujarati females were assessed to have metabolic syndrome (NCEP ATP-III) in a study sample of 840 by Gupta et al. (2004), Goa; Peixoto and Shah (2014) estimated that 39.8% of females residing in Mandur Village of North district Goa satisfied the mNCEP ATP-III criterion, Gujarat (34.6%, NCEP ATP-III) illustrated by Patel et al. (2016), Maharashtra; Mumbai females (NCEP ATP-III: 22.0%) studied by Jadhav et al. (2014), Maharashtra; among mumbai females, Sawant et al. (2011) observed the prevalence of metabolic syndrome as 12.6% according to mNCEP ATP-III guidelines, Maharashtra; Kamble et al.(2010) conducted a study in females of Wardha district of Mumbai and observed the prevalence of metabolic syndrome as 7.6% based on the NCEP ATP-III criterion and the minimum prevalence in Western region was observed in Maharashtra (7.0%, IDF) postulated by Jadhav et al. (2014).

In Eastern Region studies, the highest prevalence of MS (55.6%, IDF)was observed in the women of West Bengal illustrated by Banerjee et al. (2019) followed by women of Orissa where Prasad et al.(2012) conducted study on 307 females of Orissa and reported prevalence of 52.2% using JIS definition, Bhutia tribal females of West Bengal (52.2%, NCEP ATP-III) studied by Sarkar et al. (2006). In Assam women, a study conducted by Mahanta et al. (2017) elucidated 51.1% prevalence of metabolic syndrome as per mNCEP ATP-III (2005) criterion, West Bengal; according to NCEP ATP-III criterion, Bengali females yielded 48.4% prevalence of metabolic syndrome (Sarkar et al.(2006), Assam: a cross-sectional study carried out by Kotokey et al. (2013) diagnosed 45.9% prevalence of metabolic syndrome using IDF definition.Similarly, Srimani et al. (2017) performed an investigation among females of West Bengal and encountered 45.9% estimates of MS on the basis of IDF standard, Odisha (28.3, mNCEP ATP-III) studied by Manjareeka et al. (2018), Manipur; In Imphal state, 21.0% females ranging in age between 21-70 years met ATP-III criterion for metabolic syndrome (Rothangpui et al. 2015), West Bengal (6.0%, JIS) a study conducted by Das et al. (2017) and3.8% Toto tribal females of West Bengal diagnosed with MS as per NCEP ATP-III diagnostic criterion.

In Central Region studies, Jain et al. (2015) in their study among females of Central India reported 13.5% prevalence of metabolic syndrome as per ATP-III (2001) standard. On the other hand, 8.1% females of Indore, Madhya Pradesh met with mNCEP ATP-III criterion of MS ranging in age 20-80 years (Agrawal et al. 2017).

DISCUSSION

To our knowledge, this is the first systematic review that has investigated the prevalence of MS in India. Overall, 44 epidemiological studies have been reviewed for the prevalence of MS among female populations of India. This choice was made to allow valid comparison of studies from various regions of India. Due to the extensive heterogeneity among studies, meta-analysis was not performed. The observations of the present review provide an insight into the magnitude of the burden of MS in India.

There have been a number of studies of metabolic syndrome among females of India (Table 2). In these female populations of India, the prevalence of metabolic syndrome varied from 3.8% to 67.8% primarily due to different diagnostic criteria used for the assessment of metabolic syndrome, divergence in subject inclusion and exclusion criteria as well as sample size, urbanization level, ethnic variation, difference in the age group and socio-demographic characteristics, divergence in lifestyle habits and periodic dissimilarity of studies. Accumulating evidences from literature elucidated that most of the studies used WHO, NCEP ATP-III, IDF and mNCEP ATP-IIIdiagnostic criteria for diagnosis of metabolic syndrome.

Very few studies have assessed the prevalence of metabolic syndrome according to JIS criterion (harmonised Asian-specific guidelines). This review also revealed evidently that only one study conducted in Northern Region among females of Amritsar, Punjab applied five internationally recognized diagnostic criterion including JIS criterion (harmonised Asian-specific guidelines) to assess the prevalence of MS and screened 52.1%, 47.5%, 46.4%, 41.5% and 13.1% females with MS using JIS (2009), IDF (2005), mNCEP ATP-III (2005), NCEP ATP-III (2001) and WHO (1999) guidelines, respectively. Overall, the minimum 3.8% prevalence of MS was observed among Toto tribal females of West Bengal in Eastern Region as per NCEP ATP-III diagnostic criterion (Sarkar et al. 2006) whereas the maximum 67.8% females of Kerala in Southern Region diagnosed with MS by Vatakencherry and Saraswathy (2019). On applying NCEP ATP-III guidelines.It is apparent from the literature that till date two multicentric studies were conducted for the assessment of prevalence of MS in India. Deedwania et al. (2014) conducted a multicentric study in 11 cities of India on 2772 females aged ≥20 and reported the prevalence of MS as 22.80, 34.50% and 40.40%on applying NCEP ATP-III (2001), mNCEP ATP-III (2005) and JIS (2009) standards, respectively. Thiruvagounder (2010) also conducted a large cross-sectional study on local Indian population and reported the prevalence of MS as 27.0% in the females.

It can be concluded from the present review article that prevalence of metabolic syndrome is on the rise throughout the India due to prompt socioeconomic transitions accompanied with affluence, urbanization, mechanization, auto-mobilization, and urban migration. India has already become the diabetic capital of the world and the other non-communicable diseases are also on the rise. Metabolic syndrome is considered to be a precursor to many non- communicable diseases. In order to slow down this progression we need to conduct multi centric studies to assess the national prevalence of metabolic syndrome and to initiate remedial measures. Therefore, early identification of the metabolic abnormalities and taking appropriate intervention by instituting holistic, multidisciplinary, and multi-sectorial preventive measures at an individual, community, and societal level would help to promote healthy dietary habits and physically active lifestyles that may fight against the growing epidemic of metabolic syndrome.

ACKNOWLEDGMENTS

We would like toexpress our profound gratitude to all thefemales for their cooperation and contribution towards this study. We are whole-heartedly thankful to Miss Jaspree tKaur for her assistance in the collection of data. The authors deeply acknowledge the funding received from the Guru Nanak Dev University under the scheme University with Potential for Excellence (UPE) and Centre with Potential for Excellence in Particular Area (CPEPA).

Author Disclosure Statement: No conflicts of interest. The authors have no disclosures to make in relation to the content of this manuscript.

REFERENCES

Agrawal, J., Bharihoke, N. and Kar A. (2016). Incidence of metabolic syndrome in the urban population of Indore, Madhya Pradesh, India. *Innovare journal of Medical Sciences*5 (1): 25-28.

Alberti, K.G. and Zimmet, P.Z. (1998). Definition, diagnosis and classification of diabetes mellitus and its complications: Diagnosis and classification of diabetes mellitus provisional report of WHO consultation. *Diabet Med.* 15: 539 –53.

Alberti, K.G., Eckel, R.H., Grundy, S.M., Zimmet, P.Z., Cleeman, J.I., Donato, K.A. et al. (2009). Harmonizing the metabolic syndrome: a joint interim statement of the International Diabetes Federation Task Force on Epidemiology and Prevention; National Heart, Lung and Blood Institute; American Heart Association; World Heart Federation; International Atherosclerosis Society; and International Association for the Study of Obesity. *Circulation* 120(16): 1640-1645.

Alberti, K.G., Zimmet, P. and Shaw, J. (2006). Metabolic syndrome-a new worldwide definition. A consensus statement from the International Diabetes Federation. *Diabet Med* 23: 469-480.

Allam, R.R., Pant, R., Uthappa, C.K., Dinaker, M., Guganti, G. and Yeldandi, V.V. (2018). Prevalence of Vitamin D Deficiency, Metabolic Syndrome and Association between the Two in a South Asian Population. *J Nutr Disorders Ther* 8:2 doi: 10.4172/2161-0509.1000229.

Awosan, K.J., Ibrahim, M.T.U., Arisegi, S.A., Ejimadu, S.P., Erhiano, E.E. and Aderahman, A.T. (2013). Prevalence of metabolic syndrome and its components among civil servants in a metropolitan city in Northern Nigeria. *Global Advanced Research Journal of Medicine and Medical Sciences* 2(11): 238-246.

Banerjee, R., Dasgupta, A., Naskar, N.N., Kundu, P.K., Pan, T. and Burman, J. (2019). A study on the prevalence of metabolic syndrome and its components among adults aged 18–49 years in an urban area of West Bengal. *Indian J Indian J Community Med* 2019; 44: 261-4.

Bansal, S., Paliwal, A., Verma, V. and Chauhan, J. (2017). A study on the prevalence of metabolic syndrome in the general population in Western Uttar Pradesh, India. International *Journal of Research in Medical Sciences* 5: 2641.

Bhat, R.A., Laway, B.A. and Zargar, A.H. (2010). Prevalence of metabolic syndrome in Kashmir valley of Indian subcontinent. *Indian J Med Sci.* 64(6): 259-64.

Carr, M.C. (2003). The Emergence of the Metabolic Syndrome with Menopause. *The Journal of Clinical Endocrinology & Metabolism* 88(6): 2404–2411, https://doi.org/10.1210/jc.2003-030242.

Chinawale, C.G., Parmar, D.V., Kavathia, P., Rangnani, T., Thakkar, J. and Kartha, G. (2018). Metabolic syndrome among adults of surendranagar District of Saurashtra, Gujarat: A cross-sectional Study. *Indian J Community Med* 43: 24-8.

Cornier, M., Dabelea, D., Hernandez, T.L., Lindstrom, R.C., Steig, A.J., Stob, N.R., Van Pelt, R.E., Wang, H. and Eckel, R.H. (2008). The Metabolic Syndrome. *Endocrine Reviews* 29(7): 777– 822.

Das, T.P., Sen, M., Saha, I., Chaudhuri, D., Das, T.P., Sen, M., Saha, I. (2017) *Int J Cur Res Rev* 9(4): 14-18.

Deepa, M., Farroq, S., Datta, M., et al. (2007). Prevalence of metabolic syndrome using WHO, ATP-III and IDF definitions in Asian Indians: The Chennai urban rural epidemiology study (CURES-34). *Diabetes/ Metabolism Research and Reviews* 23: 127-134.

Expert Panel on Detection, Evaluation and Treatment of high blood cholesterol in adults. Executive Summary ogf the Third Report of the National Cholesterol Education Program (NCEP) Expert Panel on Detection, Evaluation and Treatment of high blood cholesterol in adults (ATP-III). (2001). *JAMA* 285(19): 2486-97.

Ford, E.S. (2004). Prevalence of metabolic syndrome in US populations. *Endcrinology and Metabolism Clinics of North America* 33 (2): 333-350.

Ford, E.S., Giles, W.H. and Dietz, W.H. (2002). Prevalence of metabolic syndrome among US adults: findings from the Third National Health and Nutrition Examination Survey. *JAMA* 287: 356-359.

Grundy, S.M. (2008). Metabolic Syndrome pandemic. *Arterioscler Thromb Vasc Biol.* 28(4): 629-36.

Gupta, R., Deedwania, P.C., Gupta, A., Rastogi, S., Panwar, R.B. and Kothari, K. (2004). Prevalence of Metabolic Syndrome in an Indian urban population. *International Journal of Cardiology* 97: 257-261.

Hajian-Tilaki, K. (2015). Metabolic syndrome and its associated risk factors in Iranian adults: A systematic review. *Caspian J Intern Med* 6(2): 51-61.

Harikrishnan, S., Sarma, S., Sanjay, G., Jeemon, P., Krishnan, M.N. and Venugopal, K. et al. (2018). Prevalence of metabolic syndrome and its risk factors in Kerala, South India: Analysis of a community based cross-sectional study. *PLoS One* 13: e0192372.

International Diabetes Federation (IDF, 2005). *The IDF consensus worldwide definition of the metabolic syndrome.* Available at: http://www.idf.org/webdata/ducs/ IDF_Metasyndrome definition.pdf (accessed May 2005).

Isomaa, B., Almgren, P., Tuomi, T., Forsen, B., Lahti, K., Nissen, M., Taskinen, M.R. and Groop, L. (2001). Cardiovascular morbidity and mortality associated with the metabolic syndrome. *Diabetes Care* 24: 683-689.

Jain, J., Rao, T., Desmukh, P. and Bnait, S. (2015). Prevalence and Correlates of Metabolic Syndrome in Young Population: A Cross Sectional Study. *J Diabetes Metab* 6 (3): 1-5.

Kamble, P., Deshmukh, P.R.and Garg, N. (2010). Metabolic syndrome in adult population of rural Wardha, Central India *Indian J Med Res* 132: 701-705.

Kamble, P., Deshmukh, P.R. and Garg, N. (2010). Metabolic syndrome in adult population of rural Wardha, central India. *Indian Journal of Medical Research* 132: 701-705.

Kapil U and Kaur S. (2010). Prevalence of pediatric metabolic syndrome (PMS) amongst children in the age group of 6-18 years belonging to high-income group residing in National Capital Territory (NCT) of Delhi. *Indian J Pediatr* 77: 1041.

Kaur, J. (2014). A Comprehensive Review on Metabolic Syndrome. *Cardiol Res Pract* p. 21. doi: http://dx.doi.org/10.1155/2014/943162.

Khan, Y., Lalchandani, A., Gupta, A.C., Khadanga, S. and Kumar, S. (2018). Prevalence of metabolic syndrome crossing 40% in northern India: Time to act fast before it runs out of proportions. *J Family Med Prim Care* 7: 118-23.

Kimm, M.H., Kim, M.K., Choi, B.Y. and Shin, Y.J. (2004). Prevalence of metabolic syndrome and its association with cardiovascular disease in Korea. *J Korean Med Sci* 19: 195-201.

King R.A., Rotter J.I., MotulskyA.G. Approach to genetic basis of common diseases. *Oxf Monogr Med Genet* 2002; 44: 3-17.

Lakka, H.M., Laaksonen, D.E., Lakka, T.A., Niskanen, L.K., Kumpusalo, E., Tuomilehto, J. and Salonen, J.T. (2002). The metabolic syndrome and total and cardiovascular disease mortality in middle-aged men. *JAMA* 288: 2709-2716.

Lerner, D.J. and Kannel, W.B. (1986). Patterns of coronary heart disease morbidity and mortality in the sexes: a 26-year follow-up of the Framingham population. *Am Heart J* 111: 383-390.

Lloyd-Jones, D., Adams, R., Carnethon, M., De Simone, G., Ferguson T.B. et al. (2009). Heart disease and stroke statistics—2009 update. A report from the American heart association statistics committee and stroke statistics subcommittee. *Circulation* 119: 480-486.

Mahanta, T.K., Joshi, R., Mahanta, B. and Gogoi, P. (2017). Determinants of metabolic syndrome (MetS) amongst persons living in Dibrugarh District of Assam *Clinical epidemiology and global health* 5: 52–61.

Mangat, C., Goel, N.K., Walia, D.K. et al. (2010). Metabolic syndrome: a challenging health issue in highly urbanized union territory of North India. *Diabetology and Metabolic Syndrome* 2(19): 1-8.

Manjareeka, M., Mishra, S., Nayak, P.K., Patro, S., Mishra, J. and Dash, S.C. (2018) metabolic syndrome among doctors: a pilot study from odisha. *Asian journal of Pharmaceutical and Clinical Research* 11 (10): 294-297.

Meenakshi, S., Devi, N.P., Vijayalakshmi, D.R., Prabhu, E. and Shanmugam, R.S. (2019). High Prevalence of Metabolic Syndrome among Outpatients in a Tertiary Care Centre, Tamil Nadu, India. *Journal of Krishna Institute of Medical Sciences University* 8(1): 52-60.

Mohammadbeigi, R., Fatholapour, A., Khodaverdi, S., Delpiseh, A., Khodaverdi, M. and Afkhamzadeh, A. (2011). Epidemiology of metabolic syndrome among women of reproductive age in Abhar city in western Iran. *Pakistan Journal of Medical Sciences* 27(5): 1116-1120.

Naik J.L., Reddy, K.S.N., Reddy, B.K.C., Basha, D.A. Prevalence and risk factors for metabolic syndrome in urban elderly: a community study from Tirupati, Chittoor district, Andhra Pradesh, India. *Int J Community Med Public Health* 2016; 3: 2106-11.

Owolabi, E.O., Goon, D.T., Adeniyi, O.V., Adedokun, A.O. and Seekoe, E. (2017). Prevalence and Correlates of Metabolic Syndrome among Adults Attending Healthcare Facilities in Eastern Cape, South Africa. *The Open Public Health Journal* 10: 148-159.

Padmavati, R. (2016). Metabolic Syndrome, serious mental illnesses & lifestyle. *Indian J Med Res* 143: 395-397 doi: 10.4103/0971-5916. 184280.

Pandey, S., Srinivas, M., Agashe, S. et al. (2010). Menopause and metabolic syndrome: a study of 498 urban women from western India. *Journal of Midlife Health* 1(2): 63-69.

Pathania, D., Bunger, R., Mishra, P. et al. (2013). A study to assess prevalence of metabolic syndrome and its socio-demographic risk factors in rural area of diatrict Ambala, Haryana. *Community Medicine and Health Education* 3: 226.

Peixoto, C. and Shah, H.K. (2014). Prevalence of metabolic syndrome among adult population in a rural area of Goa. *J Pub Health Med Res* 2(1): 34-37.

Pemminati, S., Adhikari, M.R.P., Pathak, R. and Rai, M.R.S.M. (2010). Prevalence of Metabolic Syndrome (METS) using IDF2005 Guidelines in a Semi Urban South Indian (Boloor Diabetes Study) Population of Mangalore *JAPI* 58: 674-677.

Prasad, D.S., Kabir, Z., Dash, A.K. and Das, B.C. (2012). Prevalence and risk factors for metabolic syndrome in Asian Indians: A community study from urban Eastern India. *J Cardiovasc Dis Res* 3: 204-11.

Ramachandran, A., Snehalatha, C., Satyavani, K., Sivasankari, S. and Vijay, V. (2003). Metabolic syndrome in urban Asian Indian adults—a population study using modified ATP III criteria. *Diabetes Research and Clinical Practice* 60: 199 –204.

Randhawa, R. and Sidhu, S. (2019). *Assessment of Metabolic Syndrome among adult females of Amritsar (Punjab).* Thesis Department of Human Genetics GNDU, Amritsar (Punjab) India 1-460 pages.

Ravikiran, M., Bhansali, A., Ravikumar, P., Bhansali, S., Dutta, P., Thakur, J.S., et al. Prevalence and risk factors of metabolic syndrome among Asian Indians: A community survey. *Diabetes Res Clin Pract* 2010; 8: 269-73.

Rosamond, W., Flegal, K., Friday, G., Furie, K., Go, A., et al. (2007) Heart disease and stroke statistics--2007 update: a report from the American

Heart Association Statistics Committee and Stroke Statistics Subcommittee. *Circulation* 115: e69- 171.

Roshni, M., Chandni, R. and Bhagyanathan, P.V. (2014). Metabolic Syndrome and the Frequency ofOccurrence of Its Components in Urban South Indian Population *British Journal of Medicine & Medical Research* 4(29): 4855-4867.

Rothangpui, Thiyam, G. and Joute, Z. (2015). Clinical profile in metabolic syndrome. *Int J Sci Rep* 1(5):220-5.

Saklayen M.G. (2018). The global epidemic of the metabolic syndrome. *Curr Hypertens Rep* 20:12.

Sarkar, P., Mahadeva, S.K., Raghunath, H., Upadhya, S. and Hamsa, M. (2016). Metabolic syndrome and its components among population of Holalu village, Karnataka. *Int J. Med Sci Public Health* 5(5): 860-865.

Sarkar, S., Das, M., Mukhopadhyay, B., Chakrabarti, C.S. and Majumder, P.P. (2006). High prevalence of metabolic syndrome & its correlates in two tribal populations of India & the impact of urbanization. *Indian J Med Res* 123: 679-686.

Sawant, A., Mankeshwar, R., Shah, S., Raghavan, R., Dhongde, G., Raje, H., D'souza, S., Subramanium, A., Dhairyawan, P., Todur, S. and Ashavaid, T. (2011). Prevalence of Metabolic Syndrome in Urban India. *Cholesterol* doi:10.1155/2011/920983.

Shalini, M., Babu, S.K.P., Murthy, S.A.G. et al. (2013). Metabolic syndrome among urban and rural women population- A cross sectional study. *Journal of Clinical and Diagnostic Research* 7(9): 1938-1940.

Sharma, M. and Mahna, R. (2012). Metabolic syndrome among Indian adults. *International Journal of Food and Nutritional Sciences* 1(1): 62-69.

Sharma, R., Sharma, R and Kumar, A. (2019). Metabolic syndrome: Prevalence (IDF & NCEP-ATP III) in Udhampur, Jammu city. *Int J Pharm Sci & Res* 10(3): 1420-25.

Singh, J., Rajput, M., Rajput, R and Bairwa, M. (2016). Prevalence and predictors of metabolic syndrome in a North Indian rural population: A community based study. *J Glob Diabetes Clin Metab* 1: 1-5.

Srimani, S., Saha, I. and Chaudhuri, D. (2017) Prevalence and association of metabolic syndrome and vitamin D deficiency among postmenopausal women in a rural block of West Bengal, India. *PLoS ONE* 12(11): e0188331. https://doi.org/10.1371.

Teli, A., Jabannavar, V., Adorno, I., Gayatri, G.S., Lampis, F and Patil, P (2019). Estimation of prevalence of metabolic syndrome among 1st year medical students of a medical college in North Karnataka, India. *Indian J Health Sci Biomed Res* 12: 174-8.

Thrivagouder, M., Khan, S. and Sheriff, D.S.: Prevalence of metabolic syndrome in a local population in India. *Biochemia Medica* 2010; 20: 249.

Vatakencherry, R.J. and Saraswathy, L. (2019) Prevalence of Metabolic syndrome among adults in a teaching hospital in Kochi, Central Kerala: A cross-sectional study. *J Family Med Prim Care* 8: 2079-83.

Venugopal V., Dongre A.R., Saravanan S. Prevalence and determinants of metabolic syndrome among the rural adult population of Puducherry. *Indian J Community Med* 2019; 44: 21-5.

Verma P., Srivastava R.K., Jain D. Association of lifestyle risk factors with metabolic syndrome components: A cross-sectional study in Eastern India. *Int J Prev Med* 2018; 9:6.

Xi, B.,He, D., Hu, Y. and Zhou, D. (2013). Prevalence of metabolic syndrome and its influencing factors among the Chinese adults: The China Health and Nutrition Survey in 2009. *Prev Med.* 57(6): 867–871.

Zafar, K.S., Pious, T., Singh, P.S., Gautam, R.K., Yadav, S.K., Singh, P. and Sharma H. (2017). Prevalence of metabolic syndrome in a rural population- a cross-sectional study from Western Uttar Pradesh, India. *Int J Res Med Sci* 5: 2223.

Zimmet, P., Magliano, D., Matsuzawa, Y., Alberti, G. and Shaw, J. (2005). The metabolic syndrome: A global public health problem and a new definition. *J. Atheroscler. Thromb.* 12: 295–300.

In: Ethnicity and Syndrome X
Editors: M. Das and K. Bose

ISBN: 978-1-53618-042-8
© 2020 Nova Science Publishers, Inc.

Chapter 7

PREVALENCE OF UNDERNUTRITION, OBESITY AND HYPERTENSION AMONG ADULT SHABARS AND MAHALIS OF BANKURA DISTRICT OF WEST BENGAL, INDIA

Shilpita Bhandari*[1], *Sadaruddin Biswas*[2,*], *PhD*, *Mihir Ghosh*[1], *PhD*, *Binoy Kumar Kuiti*[1], *PhD and Kaushik Bose*[1], *DSc

[1]Dept. of Anthropology, Vidyasagar University, Midnapore
[2]Department of Anthropology and Tribal Studies, Sidho-Kanho-Birsha University, Purulia

INTRODUCTION

In developing countries millions of people are facing double health burden of diseases associated with infection and nutrition along with the load

---

*Corresponding Author's Email: sadarbiswas@gmail.com.

of chronic non-communicable diseases (NCDs). Rapid urbanization has led to changes in daily activity, diet and lifestyle leading to non-communicable diseases like diabetes, Cardiovascular Diseases (CVDs), neuropsychiatric disorders. It has been reported that 36 million people were expired due to non-communicable diseases out of total 57 million of global deaths in 2008 (WHO 2010).

An improved health-care delivery system combined with rapid urbanization, industrialization, and changing lifestyle pattern during the past few decades resulted in a global transition of disease pattern from communicable to non-communicable diseases. Cardiovascular disorders once considered to affect only the affluent class have now been identified to effect people from all sections of the society and play an important determinant role for difference in life expectancy between indigenous and non-indigenous population across the world (Stoner 2012).

Various epidemiological studies recorded adverse cardio metabolic health status among South Asians, including Indians, owing mainly to the high prevalence of central obesity among them. However, most of these observations were based on studies conducted in a conglomerate of population without taking ethnicity of the population into consideration. Available data indicated that the cluster of different modifiable cardio-metabolic risk factors including central obesity, dyslipidemia, hyperglycemia, and hypertension vary across different ethnic groups and were dependent on extent of urbanization, lifestyle pattern, and socioeconomic and cultural factors (Pandit 2012). Therefore, it seemed important to assess cardio- metabolic risk profile of different population groups including the ethnic population of the country.

The prevalence of chronic or non-communicable disease is escalating much more rapidly in developing countries than in industrialized countries. World Health Organization estimates that non-communicable diseases will account for approximately three quarters of all deaths in the developing world by 2020 (WHO 1997). Syndrome X or Metabolic syndrome (MS) is characterized as the clustering of dyslipidemia, hypertension, hyper-insulinemia, and central obesity and that constitutes a risk factor for cardiovascular disease. Moreover, MS confers greater risk than a single factor for cardiovascular disease (Bitsori and Kafatos 2005, Eckel et al. 2005) and it is highly prevalent in the adult population worldwide, with a suggested ethnic predisposition among Asians (Yusuf et al. 2001). Obesity is a complex disorder and a major health risk factor for CVD, stroke, cancer, hypertension and diabetes which lead to early death (Flegal et al. 2013).

It has been reported that considerably large burden of this socio-economic disadvantage is found among Indian tribal populations. Undernutrition has been a major health concern among India tribal populations (Gopalan 1992, Basu et al. 1990). The Indian National Family and Health Survey (NFHS, 2005–06) reported that prevalence of undernutrition among the tribals was ranging between 47–48% (Basu et al. 1990). Earlier different studies have shown that the mortality and morbidity from chronic diseases among Indian populations is prevalent among people with a low body mass index (BMI), and thus they tend to accumulate intra-abdominal fat without developing the generalized risk of obesity, i.e., BMI>23 kg/m^2 (Ghosh et al. 2004). However, various developmental and economic activities undertaken by the state and central government agencies have allowed several tribes to lead a comparatively affluent lifestyle in varying proportions, which has made them vulnerable to various metabolic risk factors. Hypertension, a direct indicator of CVD, has been strongly implicated for the increased prevalence of overweight/obesity (Diaz 2002) and undernutrition (Galal 2002). Moreover, hypertension is the third most prevalent risk factor for the disease burden in south Asia (Lim et al. 2012).

The present study estimated the co-existence obesity, undernutrition, and hypertension, highlighted the risk for potential CVDs among two the tribes of Bankura district, West Bengal, India.

Methods and Materials

Study Area

The present cross-sectional study was conducted at ten villages (Bethuala, Maula, Kotro, Botdanga, Sagardanga, Katiyam, Bagdiha,

Rajamela, Harivanga and Gorurbasa) under Ranibandh, Chhatna and Gangajalghati blocks of Bankura district of West Bengal. The present investigation was conducted during March to April 2017. These villages are located around 15 km from Bankura town, the district headquarter and approximately 215 km from Kolkata, the state capital of West Bengal.

Bankura district has a population of 3,596,292, and the district has a population density of 523 inhabitants per square kilometer. Its population growth rate over the decade 2001-2011 was 12.64% and the district has a sex ratio of 954 females for every 1000 males, literacy rate of the district was 70.95% (Census 2011).

Ranibandh Community Development (CD) Block has an area of 428.51 km^2. This CD Block is located at 22°51′50″N 86°47′05″E and on the south-western part of the district, belongs to the hard rock area. The Block is surrounded by Khatra and Hirbandh CD Blocks on the north, Raipur on the east, Binpur II CD Block, of Paschim Medinipur district, on the south and Manbazar I, Manbazar II and Bandwan CD Blocks, of Purulia district, on the west.

Chhatna CD Block is located at 23°18′06″N86°58′58″E. It is 13 km from Bankura town on the Bankura-Purulia road. Chhatna CD Block has an area of 447.47 km^2. This block is bounded by Saltora and Gangajalghati CD Blocks on the north, Bankura II and Bankura I CD Blocks on the east, Indpur CD Block on the south and Kashipur and Hura CD Blocks, of Purulia district, on the west.

Gangajalghati CD Block is located at 23.42°N 87.12°E and it has an area of 366.47 km^2. The Block is located in the north-western part of the district. The Main Bankura Upland, of which this Block is a part, and characterized by undulating terrain with many hills and ridges. The area is having a gradual descent from the Chhotanagpur Plateau. The soil is laterite red and hard beds are covered with scrub jungle and sal (*Shorea robusta*) wood. Gangajalghati CD Block is bounded by Mejia CD Block on the north, Barjora CD Block on the east, Bankura II CD Block on the south and Chhatna and Saltora CD Blocks on the west.

The Participants

The present study was conducted among 446 adult (>18 year) participants, among them 226 were Shabars (male = 111 and female = 115). These participants were selected from six villages namely Bethuala, Maula, Kotro, Botdanga, Sagardanga and Katiyam. 220 adult (male= 102 and female=118) Mahalis were selected from four villages namely Bagdiha, Rajamela, Harivanga and Gorurbasa. The majority of the subjects were illiterate and very low-waged manual labourers belonging to low socio-economic status. Ethical considerations were guided by the Helsinki declaration (Goodyear et al. 2007). The district level and local administrative relevant authorities and the community leaders were informed about the objective of the present study. Verbal informed consent was obtained from each participant in their own language prior to each interview and measurement procedure.

Anthropometric Measurements

Anthropometric measurements of height (cm), weight (kg), circumferences (cm), skinfolds measurements (mm) and blood pressure (mm/hg) of each subject were measured by one investigator (SB), following the standard techniques (Lohman et al. 1988). Both height and circumference were recorded to the nearest 1 mm and weight to nearest 500 gm. For measuring blood pressure, digital blood pressure machine (Alfa Gold) was used. Technical errors of measurements (TEM) were computed and were found to be within acceptable limits (Ulijaszek & Kerr 1999).

The socio-economic and anthropometric data were collected in pre-tested questionnaire schedule. For all subjects, the same measuring equipments were used, which were calibrated daily for standardization to reduce bias or error.

Assessment of Nutritional Status

BMI was computed as weight (kg)/ height (m^2). Nutritional status was evaluated using internationally accepted BMI guidelines (WHO 1995). High BMI has been considered as a strong indicator of obesity and CVD in different populations. It has been also reported that low BMI was associated with hypertension (Jones et al. 1994). According to the World Health Organization (WHO) guidelines for Asian populations, individuals with BMI<18.5 kg/m^2 were considered as underweight; 18.5kg/m^2 but <23 kg/m^2as normal; 23 kg/m^2 but <27.5 kg/m^2 as overweight; 27.5 kg/m^2 as obese (WHO 2000).

Waist Height Ratio (WHtR) is more closely associated with central obesity, encompassing the adjustment to various statures (Hsieh et al. 2000, Lin et al. 2002, Sayeed et al. 2003) and overcoming the negative correlation of height to metabolic syndromes (Henriksson et al. 2001). It was noticed that mean height of Indian tribes is less than that of the mean height of the non-tribal population (Henriksson et al. 2001). WHtR may be treated as an ideal obesity measure and a strong indicator of health (Ashwell and Hsieh) in Indian tribal populations. In these present study, WHtR was classified in to four categories: (1) <0.40 as underweight;(2) 0.40 to <0.50 as normal (Peng et al. 2013); (3) 0.50 to <0.60 as high risk; and (4) 0.60 as morbidly high (Ashwell and Gibson 2009).

The body fat percentage was categorized into four categories, as underweight (10–13% for women; 2–5% for men), normal (14–24% for women; 6–17% for men), at risk or overweight (25–31% for women, 18–24% for men), and morbid/obese (>32% for women; >25% for men) (Muth 2009). Participants with blood pressure 140/90 mmHg were considered as hypertensive (James 2014).

Statistical Analysis

Statistical analyses were done using SPSS (Version 16.00) software. Descriptive statistics, such as mean and standard deviation (SD), were used for the selected anthropometric and physiological variables. The prevalence of hypertension in men, women, and the overall population were calculated. Undernutrition, overweight, BMI, WHtR, and body fat percentage were estimated.

RESULTS AND DISCUSSION

Demographic, anthropometric and physiological characteristics of Mahalis are presented in Table 1. Following table depicts that males were taller and heavier than their counterpart. Mean age was higher among males than females. Mean values of waist circumference, systolic BP, diastolic BP and BMI were higher among males than females. PBF was higher among females. Shabar males showed higher mean values of age, height, weight, waist circumference, systolic BP, diastolic BP and BMI than their counterpart. Similar to the Mahalis, the Shabar females showed higher mean value of PBF than males (table 2). Prevalence of underweight and overweight (table 3) were 43.14% and 7.84% among the Mahali males where Mahali females showed higher prevalence of underweight (63.56%). Similarly Shabar females showed higher prevalence of underweight (56.52%) than Shabar males (46.85%). It was also noticed that overall double burden were much higher among both tribes (Mahalis 59.55%; Shabar 57.96%). Table 4 depicts the prevalence of double burden based on WHtR among the studied populations. Overall Mahalis (44.09%) showed higher prevalence of double burden than Shabars (29.20%). Mahali females (53.39%) showed higher prevalence of double than males (33.33%). But Shabar males (34.23%) showed higher prevalence of double than females (24.35%).Table 5 represents the prevalence of total burden based on PBF among the studied populations. It was found that Shabars (43.48%) were more overweight or morbid than Mahalis (32.73%). Irrespective of ethnic group females (Mahalis 37.29%; 43.48%) were more overweight or morbid than males (Mahalis 27.45%; Shabar 30.63%). Table 6 depicts the prevalence of hypertension among the studied populations. It was noticed that Mahalis (17.73%) were more hypertensive than Shabars (14.6%). Mahali males (21.57%) were more hypertensive than females (14.41%), whereas Shabar females (19.13%) more hypertensive than males (9.91%).

Table. 1 Characteristic of the Mahalis

Descriptive statistics for Mahali individuals						
Anthropometric parameters	Male (N = 102)		Female (N = 118)		Total (N = 220)	
	Mean	S.D	Mean	S.D	Mean	S.D
Age (year)	36.5	14.75	34.0	12.89	35.1	13.81
Height (cm)	158.0	6.78	145.9	5.42	151.5	8.58
Weight (kg)	47.9	7.19	38.2	5.83	42.7	8.09
Waist circumference (cm)	75.3	7.24	71.0	10.87	73.0	9.59
Systolic (mm/Hg)	130.4	19.05	125.7	20.03	127.9	19.68
Diastolic (mm/Hg)	88.0	13.82	84.0	12.27	85.8	13.13
BMI (kg/m)	19.2	2.52	17.9	2.40	18.5	2.53
WHtR	0.5	0.05	0.5	0.07	0.5	0.06
PBF	15.2	3.85	23.9	3.77	19.9	5.79

Table 2. Characteristic of the Shabars

Descriptive statistics for Shabar individuals						
Anthropometric parameters	Male (N = 111)		Female (N = 115)		Total (N = 226)	
	Mean	S.D	Mean	S.D	Mean	S.D
Age (year)	37.9	16.30	36.8	16.98	37.3	16.62
Height (cm)	159.9	5.94	149.0	5.04	154.3	7.74
Weight (kg)	49.7	7.42	40.1	5.89	44.8	8.22
Waist circumference (cm)	75.2	6.36	69.5	7.24	72.3	7.40
Systolic (mm/Hg)	128.8	18.76	124.1	20.11	126.4	19.56
Diastolic (mm/Hg)	85.0	11.89	84.2	15.53	84.6	13.84
BMI (kg/m)	19.4	2.60	18.0	2.31	18.7	2.55
WHtR	0.5	0.04	0.5	0.05	0.5	0.04
PBF	15.8	4.13	24.7	4.36	20.4	6.15

Table 3. Prevalence of dual burden based on BMI among the studied populations

Ethnicity Vs BMI		Sex category				Total	%
		Male	%	Female	%		
Mahali	Underweight	44	43.14	75	63.56	119	54.09
	Normal	50	49.02	39	33.05	89	40.45
	Overweight/Obese	8	7.84	4	3.39	12	5.45
	Double burden	52	50.98	79	66.95	131	59.55
	Total	102	100	118	100	220	100
Shabar	Underweight	52	46.85	65	56.52	117	51.77
	Normal	46	41.44	49	42.61	95	42.04
	Overweight/Obese	13	11.71	1	0.87	14	6.19
	Double burden	65	58.56	66	57.39	131	57.96
	Total	111	100	115	100	226	100

Table 4. Prevalence of dual burden based on WHtR among the studied populations

Ethnicity Vs. WHtR		Sex category				Total	%
		Male	%	Female	%		
Mahali	Underweight	2	1.96	6	5.08	8	3.64
	Normal	68	66.67	55	46.61	123	55.91
	High risk	31	30.39	51	43.22	82	37.27
	Morbidly high	1	0.98	6	5.08	7	3.18
	Double burden	34	33.33	63	53.39	97	44.09
	Total	102	100	118	100	220	100
Shabar	Underweight	4	3.6	4	3.48	8	3.54
	Normal	73	65.77	87	75.65	160	70.8
	High risk	34	30.63	22	19.13	56	24.78
	Morbidly high	0	0	2	1.74	2	0.88
	Double burden	38	34.23	28	24.35	66	29.20
	Total	111	100	115	100	226	100

Our present study was conducted among adult Shabars and Mahalis of Bankura district, West Bengal to determine the prevalence of double burden in terms of CED, Hypertension and overweight. Present study revealed that prevalence of overall double burden was much higher among both tribes

(Mahalis 59.55%; Shabar 57.96%). The prevalence of double burden based on WHtR was 44.09% and 29.20% among Mahalis and Shabar respectively. It was noticed that Shabars (43.48%) were more overweight or morbid than Mahalis (32.73%). It was also observed that Mahalis (17.73%) were more hypertensive than Shabars (14.6%). Lima et al. (2012) reported that the prevalence of hypertension has become the third most important risk factor for the burden on diseases in south Asia. Global data represented that 20.6% of Indian men and 20.9% of Indian women were suffering from hypertension (Kearney et al. 2005) and present populations also showed similar trends of hypertension. The allover scenario on tribal was not much different as demonstrated a prevalence rate of 16.1% of hypertension among Indian tribes (Rizwanet al. (2014). A study from Brazil also reported that early childhood undernutrition may influence the occurrence of hypertension in adulthood (Sawayaet al. 2005) which makes it more essential to access the hypertension alongside undernutrition among the marginalized sections like the various tribal populations of our country. Previous studies have revealed hypertension as a critical adverse health outcome with undernutrition and obesity (Kotchen et al. 2008, Van der Sande et al. 2001). The findings of the present study revealed an increased prevalence of hypertension among undernourished and obese men as well as women. Women were at a higher risk of hypertension than men (Sawaya et al. 2005), which was also observed in our study among Shabar.

Along with undernutrition, the present study additionally revealed the considerably higher predominance of pre-hypertension, hypertension and WHtR based overweight which are worrying circumstances among Shabars and Mahalis of Bankura district, West Bengal. Previously, mentioned that the prevalence of CED among Shabars and Mahalis are also high as observed in most of the Indian tribes. Similar to other tribal populations, many risk factors of hypertensive like smoking, chewing tobacco, consumption of alcohol, etc. are also present among studied populations. During survey it was observed that majorities of them were labourers and engaged in heavy manual work. Concomitant to that, they often have inadequate dietary intake. Hence a considerably high prevalence of undernutrition can be expected among them but it was surprising that simultaneously presence of a high level of hypertension among them. Thus they suffer from a dual burden of high presence of undernutrition as well as hypertension and overweight. Therefore, this paradox needs further exploration. Ideally, longitudinal studies are required to fully comprehend the mechanism and an etiology behind this paradox. More investigations are required among Indian tribal populations.

Table 5. Prevalence of burden based on PBF among the studied populations

Ethnicity Vs. PBF		Sex category				Total	%
		Male	%	Female	%		
Mahali	Normal	74	72.55	74	62.71	148	67.27
	Overweight	28	27.45	40	33.9	68	30.91
	Morbid/Obese	0	0	4	3.39	4	1.82
	Total burden	28	27.45	44	37.29	72	32.73
	Total	102	100	118	100	220	100
Shabar	Normal	77	69.37	65	56.52	142	62.83
	Overweight	32	28.83	45	39.13	77	34.07
	Morbid/Obese	2	1.8	5	4.35	7	3.1
	Total burden	34	30.63	50	43.48	84	37.17
	Total	111	100	115	100	226	100

Table 6. Prevalence of hypertension among the studied populations

Ethnicity Vs. Hypertension		Sex category				Total	%
		Male	%	Female	%		
Mahali	Normal	80	78.43	101	85.59	181	82.27
	Hypertensive	22	21.57	17	14.41	39	17.73
	Total	102	100	118	100	220	100
Shabar	Normal	100	90.09	93	80.87	193	85.4
	Hypertensive	11	9.91	22	19.13	33	14.6
	Total	111	100	115	100	226	100

The present study highlighted the coexistence of undernutrion, overweight and hypertension among Shabars and Mahalis males of Bankura District, West Bengal. Cross-sectional nature is one of the major limitations of present study. Thus, it could not explore the causation behind this phenomenon.

ACKNOWLEDGMENTS

We are thankfully acknowledged to all the participants for their cooperation and help during data collection.

Conflicts of Interest

The authors declare that there are no conflicts of interest regarding the publication of this work.

REFERENCES

Ashwell M., Hsieh S. D. (2005). Six reasons why the waist-to-height ratio is a rapid and effective global indicator for health risks of obesity and how its use could simplify the international public health message on obesity. *International Journal of Food Sciences and Nutrition*. 56(5): 303/307.

Ashwell M., Gibson S. (2009). Waist to Height Ratio Is a Simple and Effective Obesity Screening Tool for Cardiovascular Risk Factors: Analysis of Data from the British National Diet and Nutrition Survey of Adults Aged 19–64 Years. *Obes Facts*. 2: 97–103.

Basu S. K., Jindal A., Kshatriya G. K. (1990). *Genetic and socio-cultural determinants of tribal health: A primitive KutiaKondh tribal group of Phulbani district, Orissa; ICMR Final Report*. NIHFW.

Bitsori M., Kafatos A. (2005). Dysmetabolic syndrome in childhood and adolescence. *Acta Paediatr*; 94:995-1005.

Census of India. *Indian Administrative Division (population and area).* http:/www.worldgazetteer.com/wg.php. Cited August 17, 2011.

Díaz M. E. (2002). Hypertension and obesity. *Journal of Human Hypertension*. 2002; 16 Suppl 1: S18–S22.

Eckel R. H., Grundy S. M., Zimmet P. Z. (2005). The metabolic syndrome. *Lancet*; 365:1415-28.

Flegal K. M., Kit B. K., Orpana H., Graubard B. I. (2012). Association of All Cause Mortality with Overweight and Obesity Using Standard Body Mass Index Categories. *JAMA*. 2013;309:7182.doi:10.1001.

Galal O. M. (2002). The nutrition transition in Egypt: obesity, undernutrition and the food consumption context. *Public Health Nutrition*. 5(1A), 141–148).

Goodyear, M. D. E., Krleza-Jeric, K. and Lemmens T. (2007). The Declaration of Helsinki, *British Medical Journal,* 335: 624-625.

GopalanC. (1992). Nutrition in developmental transition in South-East Asia. Regional Health Paper, SEARO, No. 21. *World Health Organization,* Regional Office for South-East Asia. New Delhi.

Ghosh A., Bose K., Chakravarti S., Das Chaudhuri A. B., Chattopadhyay J., Dasgupta G., Sengupta S. (2004). Central obesity and coronary risk factors. *J R SocPromot Health*. 124:86–90.

Hsieh S. D., Yoshinaga H., Muto T., Sakurai Y., Kosaka K. (2000). Health risks among Japanese men with moderate body mass index. *International Journal of Obesity*. 24, 358–362.

Henriksson K. M., Lindblad U., Agren B., Nilsson-Ehle P., Rastam L. (2001). Associations between body height, body composition and cholesterol levels in middle-aged men. The coronary risk factor study in southern Sweden. CRISS. *Eur J Epidemiol*. 17(6):521/526.

James P. A., Oparil S., Carter B. L., Cushman WC, Dennison-Himmelfarb C, Handler J, et al. (2014). Evidence- based guideline for the management of high blood pressure in adults: report from the panel members appointed to the Eighth Joint National Committee (JNC 8). *JAMA*. 311(5):507–520.

Jones D. W., Kim J. S., Andrew M. E., Kim S. J., Hong Y. P. (1994). Body mass index and blood pressure in Korean men and women: the Korean national blood pressure survey. *J Hypertens.* 12:1433–1437.

Kotchen T. A. (2008). Obesity-Related Hypertension? Weighing the Evidence. *Hypertension.*2008; 52: 801-802.

Lim S. S., Vos T., Flaxman A. D., Danaei G., Shibuya K., Adair-Rohani H., et al. (2012). A comparative risk assessment of burden of disease and injury attributable to 67 risk factors and risk factor clusters in 21 regions, 1990–2010: a systematic analysis for the Global Burden of Disease Study 2010. *Lancet.* 380:2224–2260.

Lin W. Y., Lee L. T, Chen C. Y., Lo H., Hsia H. H., Liu I. L., et al. (2002). Optimal cut-off values for obesity: using simple anthropometric indices to predict cardiovascular risk factors in Taiwan. *Int J Obes Relat Metab Disord.* 26(9):1232/1238.

Lohman, T. G., Roche, A. F. and Martorell, R. (1988). Anthropometric Standardization Reference Manual. *Human Kinetics Books*, Chicago Illinois.

Muth N. D. (2009). What are the guidelines for percentage of body fat loss? ACE Blog 2009 December 2. In *ACEblog California*. Available: https://www.acefitness.org/acefit/healthy-living-article/60/112/what-are-theguidelines-for-percentage-of/. Accessed 29January 2020.

Pandit K., Goswami S., Ghosh S., Mukhopadhyay P., Chowdhury S. (2012). Metabolic syndrome in South Asians. *Indian J EndocrinolMetab;*16:44-55.

Peng Y. G., Li Y., Guo M., Tian Y., Li X., Li S. H., et al. (2013). The optimal cut-off value of waist-to-height ratio for detecting severe central obesity and low body weight adult Chinese population. *Zhonghua Xin Xue Guan Bing Za Zhi.* 41(7):607–10.

Sawaya A. L., Sesso R., Florêncio T. M., Fernandes M. T., Martins P. A. (2005). Association between chronic undernutrition and hypertension. *Matern Child Nutr.* 1(3):155–63.

Sayeed M. A., Mahtab H., Latif Z. A, Khanam P. A., Ahsan K. A., Banu A., et al. (2003). Waist-to-height ratio is a betterobesity index than body mass index and waist-to-hip ratio for predicting diabetes, hypertension and lipidemia. *Bangladesh Med Res Counc Bull.* 29(1):1/10.

Stoner L., Stoner K. R., Young J. M., Fryer S. (2012). Preventing a cardiovascular disease epidemic among indigenous populations through lifestyle changes. *Int J Prev Med*; 3:230-39.

Ulijaszek, S.J., and Kerr, D.A. (1999).Anthropometric measurement error and the assessment of nutritional status.*British Journal of Nutrition*, 82, 165-177.

Van der Sande M. A., Ceesay S. M., Milligan P. J., Nyan O. A., Banya W. A., Prentice A., et al. (2001). Obesity and Undernutrition and Cardiovascular Risk Factors in Rural and Urban Gambian Communities. *American Journal of Public Health.* 91(10):1641–1644.

World Health Organization. (1997). *Global strategy for non-communicable disease prevention and control (draft).* Geneva, Switzerland: World Health Organization; (Publication no. WHO/NCD/GS/97.1).

WHO/IOTF/IASO (2000). *The Asia-Pacific perspective: Redefining Obesity and its Treatment. Hong Kong: World Health Organization, International Obesity Task Force*, International Association for the Study of Obesity.

World Health Organization (2010). Global status report on non-communicable diseases. Geneva: *WHO*, 2011. Available at: http://www.who.int/nmh/publications/ncd_report_full_en.pdf. Accessed 25 January 2020.

Yusuf S., Reddy S., Ounpuu S., Anand S. (2001). Global burden of cardiovascular disease: Part II: variations in cardiovascular disease by specific ethnic groups and geographic regions and prevention strategies. *Circulation;* 104:2855-64.

In: Ethnicity and Syndrome X
Editors: M. Das and K. Bose
ISBN: 978-1-53618-042-8
© 2020 Nova Science Publishers, Inc.

Chapter 8

EFFECT OF HUMAN MIGRATION ON HYPERTENSION, CARDIOVASCULAR DISEASES, TYPE 2 DIABETES AND THEIR ASSOCIATIONS WITH METABOLIC SYNDROME AMONG THE ASIAN INDIANS

Nitish Mondal[1,*] and Jaydip Sen[2]
[1]Assistant Professor, Department of Anthropology,
Assam University (Diphu Campus), Karbi-Anglong, Assam, India
[2]Professor, Department of Anthropology, North Bengal University,
Darjeeling, West Bengal, India

INTRODUCTION

The effects of migration on human health have been a topic of interest for anthropologists, demographers and human biologists. Even if migrants

* Corresponding Author's Email: nitishanth@gmail.com.

who travel to a new region so as to achieve a higher living standards in their new place of residence, the improved living conditions may not be associated with concerns of better health conditions of individual/populations (Madrigal et al., 2011). Part of the difficulties in understanding health consequences of migration are the major complications in trying to control variables that may affect the overall health status, such as sex/gender, age and urban or rural environment of migrants and non-migrants individual/populations (Madrigal et al., 2011; Kozieł et al., 2012). The effects of human migration on overall health status have received significant amount of attention from researchers and the scientific community, who have been focused on the differences in health issues, adiposity pattern (e.g., overweight, obesity and central adiposity) and related co-morbidities and mortality patterns between migrant groups on the one hand, and migrants and the native-born population on the other (e.g., Kusuma et al., 2009; Madrigal et al., 2011; Kozieł et al., 2012; Shah et al., 2015). Compared to those they leave behind, international or long-distance intra-national migrants are often relatively healthy, and this is commonly referred to as a *'healthy migrant effect.'* Therefore, moving itself can have both positive and negative implications for the health status in individuals/populations. On the positive side of human migration, especially those moving from a poor to a rich countries may have better access to healthcare services and favorable environment conditions in the new home country, and may benefit from better diets and/or a cleaner environment and health status. Since such migrants may also carry with them a health deficit from their area of origin, it might be expected that their health condition would nevertheless be worse than that of the native-born populations (e.g., Shah et al., 2015). However, new migrants may also experience certain advantages arising from their continued patterns of beliefs, practices, lifestyle and social contacts that protect them from dangers of the new environment, thus, resulting in an *'epidemiological paradox'* of better than expected health outcomes (e.g., Morales et al., 2002; Madrigal et al., 2011; Koziel et al., 2012). Given the increase in population migration both voluntary and forced all over the world and the web of interconnections between migration and health status, it might be assumed that robust theories exist which could explain the multiple relationships between migration and overall health status in *'Asian Indian'* or *'Asian phenotype'*. In an Asian setting, collaborative research investigations both by social and epidemiological researchers mainly focused on the field of communicable disease vulnerability among migrants and/or host population and also the serious manifestations of several non-communicable diseases (e.g., hypertension, type-II diabetes, cardiovascular diseases and metabolic disorders). Much of research at the intersection between human migration and health effect was reported on the developed countries where, the role of health-selective migration in explaining the widening health gap between the higher and lower socio-economic group was examined (Norman et al., 2005). Moreover, the importance of examining migration and health status needs to pay closer attention to the varied meanings of health and illness, as well as to the socio-economic, demographic and socio-cultural contexts of its relationships to human migration in Asian Indians (Boyle et al., 2003; Madrigal et al., 2011).

The population migration may have far-reaching ramifications for various animals, including humans, because migration has the potential to spread and/or emerging diseases to new geographic areas or recipient population (e.g., Li et al., 2005; Liu et al., 2005; Olsen et al., 2006). The answers to these questions are important from a scientific research standpoint, but they will also help us to determine how best to conserve or restore the desired health status of migratory populations. Many populations of migrants are declining and others are becoming more sedentary, more technologically dependent or advanced and became vulnerable due to their genetic constituents and still others may not be able to cope up due to rapid climatic change, environment and alterations in habitat (e.g., Wilcove and Wikelski 2008). Rural-to-urban migration is among the most common type of migration especially among developing countries. Current trends suggested that this is the most frequent population migration occurring from countries from low-middle income to developed nations. The data suggest that urbanization, healthcare facilities, employment, education, industrialization, socio-economic situations, urban amenities and modernization could be the major pull or determinant factors for population migration. This massive movement of the migrants has implications for the overall health of individuals and groups and they are not a homogeneous group, and their health is affected more by the conditions under which they migrated and the social and environment conditions in which they live in the receiving country (e.g., Olsen et al., 2006; Maffla, 2008; Wilcove and Wikelski 2008; Madrigal et al., 2011). The rapid transformation of the socio-economic condition, initiated at the turn of the 1980s and 1990s, has caused dramatic changes in the social structure, with massive short-distance migration, mainly from rural areas to nearby big urban and sub-urban regions. Therefore, such population mobility is advantageous for the reduction of unemployment, and further development of industrialized regions in relation to economic development (e.g., Olszewska and Łaska-Mierzejewska 2008; Szklarska et al., 2008). Several research investigations have reported the health effects of migration has largely focused on population movements between countries (e.g., McKay et al., 2003; Madrigal et al., 2011). Several researchers have already advocated that health effects of migration from rural-to-urban areas within countries is less extensive, due to the well-known driven factors of migration such as socio-economic, education, employment, healthcare facilities and other factors that are likely to be related to health. Migrants are often not representative of the rural area they come from making valid comparisons between migrants and non-migrants difficult (e.g., Miranda et al., 2011). Therefore, one is also interested in how migrants are affected by their environments—especially because humans are currently fragmenting or destroying migrants' habitats, exploiting some migratory populations, depleting resources, altering the aerosphere and changing the climate (Kunz, 2008). Migration research investigations are found to be powerful means of identifying environmental causes of common diseases as changes in environment are large and occur at a known time, making causal inferences more feasible. McKay et al. (2003) reported that it is clear that migrants in general tend to suffer from worse health and display disadvantaged risk factor profiles such cardiovascular risk factors, hypertension, diabetes and obesity. In comparison to the host population they are more frequently subject to hypertension, chronic health conditions, low birth weight, and excess adiposity or obesity in population. Moreover, their ill health and unfavourable risk profiles may worsen with increasing duration of stay. Urban-rural comparisons are of limited relevance in examining the effects of urban migration in developing countries where urbanization is due to growth of existing urban populations, expansion of urban boundaries and rural in-migration. Cultural, genetic and lifestyle backgrounds of migrants and host populations further limit the value of rural-urban comparisons in population (Lyngdoh et al., 2006; Madrigal et al., 2011). Migration affects not only the body composition of the individual/population, but also the concepts of illness and disease prevalence, modes of communication and cultural expectations and the healthcare and composition. Since the healthcare system is strongly based on processes of social interaction, questions arise as to how its various healthcare providers cope with the cultural and ethnic diversity of their migrants in host populations.

STATEMENT OF HEALTH PROBLEM AND OBJECTIVES OF THE PRESENT REVIEW

Urbanization is an important demographic phenomenon throughout the globe, and it transforms the human settlement pattern from rural areas to predominantly urban regions. Since time, such demographic transformation has increased the profound effects on the biological and social issues among human population. Understanding the biological consequences of this change in settlement pattern is an important challenge for human biologists, biological anthropologist and demographers. One approach to understanding the effects of urban environments on human biology has been to investigate rural-to-urban migrants. The population migration pattern is generally very complex in nature and, migrants have the propensity to migrate from the rural habitats to experience an urban environment of large settlements, extraordinarily heterogeneous environments with enormous socio-economic differentials in health condition. Environment conditions of the urban areas have the main hazards of different biological, social and lifestyle related issues among the migrants. Such differences in the environment have created a change in the lifestyle, disease and health status of the migrants. Young migrants from the distant places are generally healthy, but the existing literature search has clearly highlighted the issues that disease prevalence and health status is differing considerably among migrants than non-migrants. Therefore, the objectives of the present review study are to understand the current conditions, causes and effects in rural-to-urban migration on the disease prevalence and health issues among adult Asian Indian migrants of low-middle income countries. Many investigations have reported relationships between health and migration, which are modified by age and migration distance (Kusuma et al., 2009; Madrigal et al., 2011). Researchers have shown that changes in correlations between health status and migration occur independently of age, stage of life, migration distance and reasons for migration. Thus, depending on the reasons for migration, migrants can be more or less healthy than their non-migrant counterparts. The relationship between migration and poor health status is clearly visible in the case of mental illness. The suggestion that migration can contribute to an increase or decrease in place-specific rates of illness is not new. However, differences in health status between small geographical locations that may be affected by the inter-relationships between health, area-based deprivation and migration are under-researched (Norman et al., 2005). The present review study also discusses the effects of human migration on hypertension, cardio-vascular diseases, type-II diabetes and their associations with metabolic syndrome among Asian Indians.

HYPERTENSION

Human migration (e.g., rural-to-urban) provides an ideal opportunity to examine the effects of environment and genetic predisposition and susceptibility on blood pressure and/or prevalence hypertension in individuals/population. The prevalence of higher awareness, treatment, and control rates, for both hypertension and diabetes were observed in rural-to-urban migrants and urban participants compared with rural participants or non-migrants individuals (e.g., Madrigal et al., 2011; Lerner et al., 2013; Dastan et al., 2017; Bernabe-Ortiz et al., 2017; Leyvraz et al., 2018). Migration studies revealed that increased sodium consumption is a key factor for the development of hypertension in some ethnic group/population, and people are known to be more prone to develop hypertension in developed countries. Rural-urban migration coupled with acculturation, modernization and urbanization trends have significant relationship with the development of high blood pressure or hypertension among low-middle income countries (e.g., Bernabe-Ortiz et al., 2017). Conversely, for some common causes of chronic disease in the country of origin, environmental changes associated with migration may result in higher risks of hypertension, higher Body Mass Index (BMI), obesity and cardio-vascular diseases (Gushulak and MacPherson, 2006; Madrigal et al., 2011; Bernabe-Ortiz et al., 2017). Research investigations have shown that the rural-to-urban migrants more often suffer from hypertension than city-dwellers do, and longer time migrants have lived in rural areas, the higher the systolic blood pressure. Thus rural environments may have detrimental effects on health of the individuals and researchers have reported that the magnitude or risk of developing hypertension was observed to higher among rural groups than urban individuals (e.g., Bernabe-Ortiz et al., 2017). Migration is considered to be a selective process and its selectivity is related to health. Several researchers have reported that young migrants, especially those moving longer distances, have shown to be healthy relative to non-migrants counterparts in population (e.g., Kusuma et al., 2009). Human migration amongst elderly people takes place among those in poor health moving to avoid environmental hazards, or to be better placed to receive care. The prevalence of excessive smoking, alcohol abuse and others unhealthy behaviours may be self-selective factors of rural-to-urban migration. A high prevalence of unhealthy behaviours such as smoking, physical inactivity and obesity have been found among migrants thus may increase the risk of hypertension (Dastan et al., 2017). Such unhealthy behaviors, among them risk factors may leads to coronary disease among many migrant groups may be a lifestyle remnant from their country or place of birth (Bernabe-Ortiz et al., 2017). A significant difference between migrants and non-migrants was detected in the rates of change of both systolic and diastolic pressures in men, and rates of change of diastolic pressures in women. Moreover, the gender specific prevalence of obesity and hypertension was observed to be higher among women than men migrant population (e.g., Madrigal et al., 2011). The urban residence and migration to urban areas can be a leading cause of increased prevalence of hypertension and the neo-migrants were subjected to more lifestyle insults and the stress generated during the adjustment process may be contributing to rise of blood pressure even at younger ages in Delhi, India (Kusuma et al., 2009).

Several researchers have reported considerable regional differences (e.g., rural-urban) in adverse health status even when demographic and socio-economic differences between those populations have been accounted in many countries (Agyemang et al., 2006; Dastan et al., 2017). Rural-urban health differences could be a cumulative result of various factors working throughout life and the longer a migrant lives in a rural area, the more health problems they accumulate, and in effect greater the differences with regard to urban dwellers. The environment influences every aspect of life, socio-economic conditions, health and well-being: housing circumstances, air quality, food and water, working conditions, distance to health care centres and mental stress due unban environment and nature of experiences of migration (Madrigal et al., 2011; Bernabe-Ortiz et al., 2017). Researchers have reported significant differences in prevalence of hypertension between populations residing in urban and rural individuals (Agyemang et al., 2006; Dastan et al., 2017). Therefore, the rural-to-urban migration has increased the relative risk of adverse health issues (e.g., hypertension) among individuals (Bernabe-Ortiz et al., 2017). Urban and rural environments differ not only with respect to population characteristics and natural surroundings, but also in terms of economic, social and cultural factors. Poor diets with low standards of hygiene are considered to have important reasons for the poor biological, physical, emotional and intellectual growths in population (Erem et al., 2009). These unhealthy behaviors may persistent in the urban environment that new migrants face, resulting in differences in health parameters between migrants and urban-dwellers. However, effect of smoking on blood pressure and its precise nature is still unclear but remains significant in population (Erem et al., 2009; Okubo et al., 2014). The association between increased alcohol consumption and blood pressure was observed to be more evident in population (Kaplan 1995; Erem et al., 2009). Thus, the elevated alcohol consumption might be responsible for much of the hypertension and higher blood pressure found among recent migrants in population. Thus, unhealthy behavior could still have continued in a new urban environment, resulting in migrant sedentary differences in health parameters like blood pressure (Kaplan 1995).

CARDIOVASCULAR DISEASES

Urbanization is occurring at a fast rate in the Low- to-Middle Income Countries (LMIC), which may be associated with less physical activity, poorer nutritional habits, and rapidly growing prevalence of cardiovascular risk factors and cardiovascular disease (CVD) with several other non-communicable diseases in Asian Indians. It is attributed that rural-to-urban migration is one of the key larger drivers of urbanization in LMIC. Thus, the evaluation of the impact of rural-to-urban migration on cardio-vascular risk factors is found to be relevant due to its huge public health consequences and economic burden in populations. With improvements in the socio-economic situation, an increasing prevalence of cardiovascular and metabolic syndrome risk factors is becoming very frequent in developing countries including South Asia (Misra et al., 2005). The magnitude was observed to be higher among particularly vulnerable population groups such as women, children, and intra-country and inter-country migrants. The main causes are increasing urbanization, nutrition transition, reduced physical activity, and genetic predisposition (Misra et al., 2005; Miranda et al., 2011; Misra and Bhardwaj, 2014). The prevalence of chronic non-communicable diseases such includes cardio-vascular diseases and metabolic disorders risk factors have increased the overall disease burden and generally accepted to be a growing concern among urban populations in LMIC (Anderson and Chu, 2007; Miranda et al., 2008). A recent consensus statement highlighted the need for data on the impact of urbanization on chronic diseases (e.g., cardio-vascular diseases and metabolic syndrome) but, such disease manifestation are growing much faster rate and increases incidence in urban areas than rural areas, partly through population migration from rural-to-urban areas (Patel and Burke, 2009; Miranda et al., 2011). It is hypothesized that insulin resistance is postulated as a central feature of the metabolic syndrome, culminating in type-II diabetes, atherosclerotic vascular disease and cardio-vascular diseases; a pathway potentially accelerated by migration/ urbanization in populations (Barnett et al., 2006). Several research investigations have clearly suggested that the early rural-to-urban migration has potential to increases the elevated risk factor of cardio-vascular diseases and metabolic risk factors among the adult migrants in both developed and developing countries. The research findings have also suggested that the age of migration and risk factors also have significantly the positive associations (Mirranda et al., 2011) and early age of migration observed to have significant effect to develop cardio-vascular diseases manifestation and metabolic syndrome risks among migrants (Misra et al., 2005; Mirranda et al., 2011). It is evident that migrant populations (i.e., rural to urban), those who migrated when aged older than 12 years had higher odds of type-II diabetes, impaired fasting glucose and metabolic syndrome compared to people who migrated at younger ages in Peru (Miranda et al., 2011).

Several research investigations have observed significant associations between human migration and cardiovascular risk factors and metabolic disorder risks (e.g., metabolic syndrome) in different ways among men and women (Misra et al., 2005). Some of the sex/gender differences could be explained by dietary differences among male and female migrants and non-migrants, or in the case of HDL cholesterol by a different association with the consumption of seal meat for men and women, but a large unexplained residual remained. Overall cardiovascular risk was higher among migrant than non-migrant males, while for women some risk factors were better and some worse among the migrants (Bjerregaard et al., 2007). In rural-urban migrants, there was a significant correlation of duration of migration with waist size, waist-to-hip ratio and systolic blood pressure. Association of risk factors with migration remained significant, though attenuated, after adjustment for socio-economic, lifestyle and obesity variables. Several researchers have also reported the effect of gender/sex related prevalence in cardio-vascular diseases among migrants' adult individuals (Bjerregaard et al., 2007; Gupta et al., 2012). The comparison of the relative risks of cardio-vascular disease with rural women, rural-urban migrants and urban have significantly greater cardio-metabolic risk factors. Prevalence is lower among urban-rural migrants. It is attributed to the gender-specific difference could be explained by differences in the dietary consumption among male and female migrants and non-migrants, or in the case of HDL cholesterol by a different association with the consumption of specific food, but a large unexplained residual remained in population (Bjerregaard et al., 2007). There is significant correlation of duration of migration with obesity and blood pressure or hypertension in adults and the differences are attenuated after adjusting for social and lifestyle variables (Gupta et al., 2012). Research investigations have shown that Asian Indian immigrants living in United States (e.g., Misra et al., 2005) as well as those living in Indian (e.g., Mohan et al., 2005), it was observed that physical inactivity was highly associated with the metabolic syndrome phenotypes. Although, at what intensity activity may be of benefit in reducing the risk of metabolic syndrome is not yet clearly understood, but one aspect is clear that active lifestyle could curb this epidemic of obesity related metabolic disorders.

TYPE-II DIABETES

Prevalence of type-II diabetes has sharply increased in most Asian countries during the last decade. This health issue has also relevant implications for the developed countries, where different research investigations have consistently revealing higher prevalence of type-II diabetes and major CVD risk factors among individuals migrating and/or originating from Asian countries than among their native populations (Barnett et al., 2006; Islam et al., 2014; Meeks et al., 2016; Modesti et al., 2016; Mishra et al., 2019). Recent data has also shown that India has one of the highest burdens of type-II diabetes worldwide, and prevalence of type-II diabetes was observed to be higher among Asian Indian immigrants that have migrated into the developed countries (Islam et al., 2014). Human migration from rural areas contributes to urbanization and increases the relative risks and prevalence of diabetes (e.g., type-II diabetes) and obesity (both central/subcutaneous and regional adiposity). The available literature review has reported that rural-to-urban migrants were observed to have a higher prevalence of obesity and type-II diabetes than rural non-migrants and that migrants would have an intermediate prevalence of obesity compared with life-long urban and rural dwellers, and that longer time since migration would be associated with a higher prevalence of type-II diabetes (e.g., Ebrahim et al., 2010). Studies have already confirmed greater prevalence of type-2 diabetes and cardiovascular disease risks in south Asians migrants in United Kingdom or Europe, that they have an increased susceptibility of developing insulin resistance in response to certain environmental conditions (e.g., urbanization), including obesity and adoption of the western or sedentary lifestyle (Barnett et al., 2006; Meeks et al., 2016). The increasing prevalence of type-II diabetes in both urban and rural population is clearly indicated that the process of urbanization is an important but not a sufficient explanation. Moreover, examination of the experiences of rural-to-urban migrants would help understand what is driving these trends in population. Several conditions are experienced by the migrants moving from poverty-ridden rural areas in early life to obesogenic urban environments in their later life. These include relative risk of excess adiposity (e.g., obesity) and type-II diabetes among both intra- and inter country migrants (Girardia et al., 2017). Tenkorang et al. (2017) reported that there was significant attenuation in their risks of type-II diabetes after accounting for lifestyle factors among women belonging to South-Asian origins. The findings were strikingly different for immigrant men, but their risks of developing type-II diabetes increased after accounting for lifestyle factors. Furthermore, it is advocated that the prevalence of type-II diabetes and cardio-vascular diseases occurred during the early age groups causes' high prevalence of premature mortality and morbidity among South-Asian populations (Gholap et al., 2011; Mishra et al., 2019).

Migrants would be expected to acquire the higher risks of the urban population if the disease is largely environmentally determined and for such trends to be dependent on the duration of time spent in a new environment and the extent to which traditional ways of living are lost—as seen for coronary heart diseases among the Japanese moving to the United States and such manifestations are generally attributed to being the westernization of lifestyle, particularly the reduction in the level of physical activity, conversion/modification to the food habits containing markedly more animal fat, simple carbohydrates, and less complex carbohydrates (Hara et al., 1996; Nakanishi et al., 2004). Several researchers have advocated that nutrition and lifestyle transition (e.g., rural-urban) had major roles to play in disclosing the predisposition for the development of type-II diabetes and great interest is now shown toward the possibility to intervene with lifestyle intervention on at risk in migratory populations (Nakanishi et al., 2004; Islam et al., 2014; Modesti et al., 2016; Girardia et al., 2017). Nakanishi et al., (2004) also reported that the prevalence of type-II diabetes and the prevalence of mortality of ischemic heart disease among Japanese-American diabetic individuals were found higher among Japanese-Americans. Furthermore, research investigations have also reported that the serum fasting insulin level as well as the insulin level after a glucose load, was higher among Japanese-Americans, even when the serum glucose levels were not statistically different as compared to native Japanese. The prevalence of obesity, which leads to insulin resistance, is higher in Japanese-Americans than that in Japanese, and that insulin resistance which is associated with type-II diabetes, hypertension, and dyslipdaemia could increase macroangiopathy such as ischemic heart disease and stroke in Japanese-Americans (Hirano et al., 2010).

METABOLIC DISORDERS

The metabolic syndrome/disorder is defined as a cluster of cardio-metabolic abnormalities that increases an individual's risk of non-insulin dependent diabetes mellitus or type-II diabetes mellitus and cardio-vascular disease. It is generally considered that the collection of central obesity or truncal obesity (e.g., abdominal/visceral adiposity), decreased high density lipoprotein cholesterol (HDL), elevated triglycerides, high blood pressures, and hyperglycemia is known as metabolic syndrome (Zimmet et al., 2005). It is estimated that a person with metabolic syndrome/disorder is essentially observed to have twice the risk for cardio-vascular diseases as compared to those without the syndrome. The development of metabolic syndrome mainly depends on individuals weight gain with body fat/adipose tissue accumulation and a predisposition to locate adipose tissue in intra-abdominal sites (e.g., visceral adiposity), including ectopic fat or within cell deposition of triglycerides in liver, pancreas and heart (Alberti et al., 2006). Moreover, it is strongly linked to a lifestyle characterized by an easy access to unlimited supply of high caloric, low nutrient-dense foods and physical inactivity (French et al., 2001). Researchers have reported that the associations of insulin resistance, which is the more commonly link with metabolic syndrome, leads to glucose metabolism disorders, dyslipidemia, high blood pressure, endothelial dysfunction, and inflammation induced by cytokine imbalance (e.g., Haslam and James, 2005). Furthermore, individuals with metabolic syndrome or type-II diabetes exhibit a characteristic pattern of abnormalities in serum lipids: low levels of HDL and elevated triglycerides. It is believed that this complex dyslipidemia, which is termed atherogenic dyslipidemia, diabetic dyslipidemia, or dyslipidemia of insulin resistance, reflects underlying insulin resistance and plays a key role in the increased cardio-vascular disease risks with type-II diabetes in individuals/population.

Several researchers worldwide on migrants have shown that Asian Indians have an increased risks of developing type-II diabetes related metabolic disorders compared to other ethnic groups and considered to be main cause of high mortality and morbidity worldwide (Kurpad et al., 2011; Das et al., 2017; Soares and Müller 2017; Mishra et al., 2019). Furthermore, the recent nutritional trends have reported that the magnitude of obesity/central obesity and the metabolic syndrome are rapidly increasing among Indian population and other south Asian countries. These are leading to increased morbidity and mortality due to metabolic disorders, type-II diabetes and cardiovascular disease (e.g., Misra and Khurana, 2009; Kurpad et al., 2011). Genetic predispositions, environmental conditions, genotype and epigenetic modification in utero remian the main causes of these physiological conditions among Asian Indians or Asian Phenotypes (e.g., Kurpad et al., 2011; Das et al., 2017; Mishra et al., 2019). Studies have reported that migration from rural areas to urban slums in a metropolitan city in India have led to high obesity, glucose intolerance and dyslipidaemia. Several factors include genetic factors and pre-migration history (e.g., socio-economic level, lifestyle habits, exposure to infections), as well as the quality of healthcare in the countries of destination controls the link between migration and prevalence of disease (e.g., metabolic disorders or type-II diabestes) (Kurpad et al., 2011; Montesi et al., 2016; Girardi et al., 2017; Mishra et al., 2019). Moreover, there are many factors (viz., urbanization, mechanization, changes in nutrition and lifestyle including physical inactivity, genetic environment/susceptibility interactions and stress) which expose the migrants to a higher risk of developing certain diseases after arrival in the host countries (Montesi et al., 2016; Das et al., 2017; Girardi et al., 2017). Several conditions experienced by migrants moving from a poverty-ridden rural area in early life to an obesogenic urban environment, positive energy gain and sedentary lifestyle in their later life increases the risk of obesity and type-II diabetes among both inter- and intra-country migrants in developed and developing countries (Kurpad et al., 2011; Girardia et al., 2017). The adoption of sedentary lifestyles and availability and abundance of calorie- dense/low fibre foods is associated with increased risks of morbidity and mortality among the migrated populations. Several researchers have also reported that population migration itself contribute to the increase in subcutaneous/abdominal or regional adiposity or obesity, hypertension and type-II diabetes with metabolic syndrome/disorders which is also an observed phenomena in Asian Indians and South Asians (Das et al., 2017; Girardi et al., 2017; Mishra et al., 2019).

CONCLUSION

Population migration causes the overall health burden by increases risks of certain non-communicable diseases and influences the epidemiology of certain diseases globally and in nations receiving migrant's population. The reduction of risk of chronic diseases (e.g., cardiovascular diseases, metabolic disorders and type-II diabetes) among rural-to-urban migrants in LMICs presents one of the major challenges to public health in the 21stcentury. The health conditions of these migrants are affected by the process of human migration in various-positive as well as negative-ways and epidemiological research could help to reveal the health inequalities between migrants and the majority population as well as to identify causes of disease and health issues. The high prevalence of obesity and genetic predisposition, urbanization, adoption western lifestyle or sedentary lifestyle and dietary modifications (e.g., cereal based diet) has increased the relative risks of non-communicable diseases among adult migrants. Therefore, appropriate health education and lifestyle modifications or intervention strategies are necessary to reduce the increased burden of such chronic diseases (e.g., hypertension, cardiovascular disease risk factors, metabolic disorders and type-II diabetes) associated with rural-urban migration among Asian Indian or Asian phenotypes. Moreover, there are possible variations seen in the environment, lifestyle, nutritional status and dietary modifications among the migratory individuals or population, therefore, an approach directed to the community rather than to the individual might, however, be more effective to reduce the overall health and disease burden in the population. Hence, specific attention is also drawn to the role of novel risk factors and cultural and socio-economic factors on occurrence and outcomes of these chronic non-communicable diseases in the population. Moreover, in order to reduce the present and future health challenges related to human migration may be more effectively addressed through collaborative global undertakings in populations. The manuscript will be helpful to understand the policy makers to introduce appropriate lifestyle intervention strategies and necessary involvement of the migrants' individuals/populations.

ACKNOWLEDGMENTS

The author gratefully acknowledged the extended help, cooperation and providing logistics support of Department of Anthropology, Assam University (Diphu Campus), Assam, India and Department of Anthropology, North Bengal, University, West Bengal, India.

REFERENCES

Agyemang C. Rural and urban differences in blood pressure and hypertension in Ghana, West Africa. *Public Health.* 2006 Jun; 120(6): 525-33. Epub 2006 May 8.

Alberti KG, Zimmet P, Shaw J. 2006. Metabolic syndrome – a new world-wide definition. AConsensus Statement from the International Diabetes Federation. *Diabetes Medicine* 23: 469–480.

Anderson GF, Chu E. Expanding Priorities −Confronting Chronic Disease in Countries with LowIncome. *N Engl J Med.* 2007; 356(3):209–11.

Barnett AH, Dixon AN, Bellary S, Hanif MW, O'hare JP, Raymond NT, Kumar S. Type 2 diabetesand cardiovascular risk in the UK south Asian community. *Diabetologia.* 2006; 49(10):2234-46.

Bernabe-Ortiz A, Sanchez JF, Carrillo-Larco RM, Gilman RH, Poterico JA1, Quispe R1, Smeeth L,Miranda JJ.Rural-to-urban migration and risk of hypertension: longitudinal results of the PERU MIGRANT study. *J Hum Hypertens.* 2017 Jan; 31(1):22-28. doi: 10.1038/jhh.2015.124. Epub 2016 Feb 11.

Bjerregaard P, Jørgensen ME, Borch-Johnsen K. Cardiovascular risk amongst migrant and non-migrant Greenland Inuit in a gender perspective. *Scand J Public Health.* 2007;35(4):380-6.

Boyle P, Graham E, Yeoh B. 2003. Editiorial introduction: labour migration and the family in Asia. *International Journal of PopulationGeography* 9(6). https://doi.org/10.1002/ijpg.311

Das A, Ambale-Venkatesh B, Lima JA, Freedman JE, Spahillari A, Das R, Das S, Shah RV, Murthy VL. Cardiometabolic disease in South Asians: A global health concern in an expanding population. *Nutr Metab Cardiovasc Dis.* 2017 Jan; 27(1):32-40. doi: 10.1016/j.numecd.2016.08.001. Epub 2016 Aug 6.

Ebrahim S, Kinra S, Bowen L, Andersen E, Ben-Shlomo Y, Lyngdoh T, Ramakrishnan L, Ahuja RC, Joshi P, Das SM, Mohan M, Davey Smith G, Prabhakaran D, Reddy KS; Indian Migration Study group. The effect of rural-to-urban migration on obesity and diabetes in India: a cross-sectional -study. *PLoS Med.* 2010;7(4):e1000268. doi: 10.1371/journal.pmed.1000268.

Gholap N, Davies M, Patel K, Sattar N, Khunti K. Type 2 diabetes and cardiovascular disease in South Asians. *Prim Care Diabetes.* 2011 Apr; 5(1):45-56. doi: 10.1016/j.pcd.2010.08.002. Epub 2010 Sep 25.

Erem C, Hacihasanoglu A, Kocak M, Deger O, Topbas M. Prevalence of prehypertension and hypertension and associated risk factors among Turkish adults: Trabzon Hypertension Study. *J Public Health* (Oxf). 2009 Mar; 31(1):47-58. doi: 10.1093/pubmed/fdn078. Epub 2008 Sep 30.

French SA, Story M and Jeffery RW. 2001. Environmental influences on eating and physical activity. *Annu Rev Public Health.*22: 309–335.

Girardi E, Schepisi MS, Goletti D, Bates M, Mwaba P, Yeboah-Manu D, Ntoumi F, Palmieri F, Maeurer M, Zumla A, Ippolito G. 2017. The global dynamics of diabetes and tuberculosis: the impact of migration and policy implications. *Int J Infec Diseases.* 56:45-53.

Gupta R, Gupta R, Agrawal A, Misra A, Guptha S, Pandey RM, Misra P, Vikram NK, Dey S, Rao S, Menon VU, Kamalamma N, Revathi K, Mathur B, Sharma V. Migrating husbands and changing cardiovascular risk factors in the wife: a cross sectional study in Asian Indian women. *J Epidemiol Community Health.* 2012;66(10):881-9. doi: 10.1136/jech-2011-200101. Epub 2011 Dec 6.

Gushulak BD, MacPherson DW. 2006. The basic principles of migration health: population mobility and gaps in disease prevalence. *Emerg Themes Epidemiol* 3:3.

Hara H, Egusa G, Yamakido M. Incidence of non-insulin-dependent diabetes mellitus and its risk factors in Japanese-Americans living in Hawaii and Los Angeles. *Diabet Med.* 1996;13(9 Suppl6):S133-42.

Haslam DW, James WP. 2005. Obesity. *Lancet.*366:1197-209.

Hirano M, Nakanishi S, Yamane K. *Macroangiopathy compared between native Japanese and Japanese-Americans: Findings from the Hawaii-Los Angels-Hiroshima Study*. Nihon Rinsho. 2010;68(5):857-60.

Islam NS, Zanowiak JM, Wyatt LC, Kavathe R, Singh H, Kwon SC, Trinh-Shevrin C. 2014. Diabetes prevention in the New York City Sikh Asian Indian community: a pilot study. *Int J Environ Res PublicHealth.* 2014 May 19;11(5):5462-86. doi: 10.3390/ijerph110505462.

Kaplan NM. Alcohol and Hypertension. *Lancet* 345: 1588.

Kozieł S, Lipowicz A, Ulijaszek SJ. 2012. Detrimental effects of early rural life on blood pressure among urban male migrants in Wrocław, Poland. *Anthropological Review* 75(2):83-91.

Kunz R. Globalisation and Migration: New Issues, New Politics? *Third World Quarterly* Vol. 29, No. 7, (2008), pp. 1389-1409

Kurpad AV, Varadharajan KS, Aeberli I. The thin-fat phenotype and global metabolic disease risk. *Curr Opin Clin Nutr Metab Care.* 2011 Nov; 14(6):542-7. doi: 10.1097/MCO.0b013e32834b6e5e.

Kusuma Y, Gupta S, Pandav C. Migration and hypertension: a cross-sectional study among neo-migrants and settled-migrants in Delhi, India. *Asia Pac J Public Health.* 2009; 21(4):497-507. doi: 10.1177/1010539509344114.

Kusuma Y, Gupta S, Pandav C. Migration and hypertension: a cross-sectional study among neo-migrants and settled-migrants in Delhi, India. *Asia Pac J Public Health.* 2009 Oct; 21(4):497-507. doi: 10.1177/1010539509344114.

Lerner AG, Bernabe-Ortiz A, Gilman RH, Smeeth L, Miranda JJ. The "rule of halves" does not apply in Peru: awareness, treatment, and control of hypertension and diabetes in rural, urban, and rural-to-urban migrants. *Crit Pathw Cardiol.* 2013; 12(2):53-8. doi: 10.1097/HPC.0b013e318285ef60.

Leyvraz M, Mizéhoun-Adissoda C, Houinato D, MoussaBaldé N, Damasceno A, Viswanathan B, Amyunzu-Nyamongo M, Owuor J, Chiolero A, Bovet P. Food Consumption, Knowledge, Attitudes, and Practices Related to Salt in Urban Areas in Five Sub-Saharan African Countries. *Nutrients.* 2018 Aug 7;10(8). pii: E1028. doi: 10.3390/nu10081028.

Li L, Wang HM, Ye XJ, Jiang MM, Lou QY, Hesketh T. The mental health status of Chinese rural-urban migrant workers : comparison with permanent urban and rural dwellers. *Soc Psychiatry Psychiatr Epidemiol.* 2007;42(9):716-22.

Lu Y. Rural-urban migration and health: evidence from longitudinal data in Indonesia. *Soc Sci Med.* 2010; 70(3):412-9. doi: 10.1016/j.socscimed.2009.10.028.

Lyngdoh T, Kinra S, Shlomo YB, Reddy S, Prabhakaran D, Smith GD, Ebrahim S; Indian migration study group. Sib-recruitment for studying migration and its impact on obesity and diabetes. *Emerg Themes Epidemiol.* 2006;3:2.

Madrigal L, Brady J, Raxter M, Ruiz E, Otarola F, Blell M. Obesity, hypertension, and migration: a meta-analysis of populations of the South Asian diaspora. *Hum Biol.* 2011; 83(1):71-86. doi: 10.3378/027.083.0105.

Maffla C. Health in the age of migration: migration and health in the EU. *Community Pract.* 2008 Aug;81(8):32-5.

McKay, L.; Macintyre, S.; Ellaway, A. *Migration and health: a review of the international literature.*

Medical Research Council, *Social & Public Health Sciences Unit,* University of Glasgow; Glasgow: 2003. Occasional paper No. 12.

Miranda JJ, Gilman RH, Smeeth L. Differences in cardiovascular risk factors in rural, urban and rural-to-urban migrants in Peru. *Heart.* 2011;97(10):787-96. doi: 10.1136/hrt.2010.218537.

Miranda JJ, Kinra S, Casas JP, Smith G Davey, Ebrahim S. Non-communicable diseases in low- and middle-income countries: context, determinants and health policy. *Trop Med Int Health.* 2008; 13(10):1225–34.

Mishra SR, Ghimire S, Joshi C, Gyawali B, Shrestha A, Neupane D, Sharma SR, Pokharel Y, Virani SS. Cardio-metabolic disease risk factors among South Asian labour migrants to the Middle East: a scoping review and policy analysis. *Global Health.* 2019 May 2; 15(1):33. doi: 10.1186/ s12992-019-0468-8.

Misra A, Khurana L. The metabolic syndrome in South Asians: epidemiology, determinants, and prevention. *Metab Syndr Relat Disord.* 2009 Dec;7(6):497-514. doi: 10.1089/met.2009.0024.

Misra A1, Bhardwaj S. Obesity and the metabolic syndrome in developing countries: focus on South Asians. *Nestle Nutr Inst Workshop Ser.* 2014; 78:133-40. doi: 10.1159/000354952. Epub 2014 Jan 27.

Misra KB, Endemann SW, Ayer M. 2005. Leisure time physical activity and metabolic syndrome in Asian Indian immigrants residing in northern California. *Ethn Dis.*15:627-634.

Mohan V, Gokulakrishnan K, Deepa R et al., 2005. Association of physical inactivity with components of metabolic syndrome and coronary artery disease—the Chennai Urban Population Study (CUPS no. 15). *Diabet Med.* 22: 1206-1211.

Montesi L, Caletti MT, Marchesini G. 2016. Diabetes in migrants and ethnic minorities in a changing World. *World J Diabetes.* 7:34–44.

Morales LS, Lara M, Kington RS, Valdez RO, Escarce JJ. Socioeconomic, cultural, and behavioral factors affecting Hispanic health outcomes. *J Health Care Poor Underserved.* 2002 Nov; 13(4):477-503.

Nakanishi S, Okubo M, Yoneda M, Jitsuiki K, Yamane K, Kohno N. A comparison between Japanese-Americans living in Hawaii and Los Angeles and native Japanese: the impact of lifestyle westernization on diabetes mellitus. *Biomed Pharmacother.* 2004;58(10):571-7.

Norman P, Boyle P, Rees P. Selective migration, health and deprivation: a longitudinal analysis. *Soc Sci Med.* 2005; 60(12):2755-71.

Okubo Y, Sairenchi T, Irie F, Yamagishi K, Iso H, Watanabe H, Muto T, Tanaka K, Ota H. Association of alcohol consumption with incident hypertension among middle-aged and older Japanese population: the Ibarakai Prefectural Health Study (IPHS). *Hypertension.* 2014 Jan; 63(1):41-7. doi: 10.1161/HYPERTENSIONAHA.113.01585. Epub 2013 Oct 14.

Olsen B, Munster VJ, Wallensten A, Waldenström J, Osterhaus AD, Fouchier RA. Global patterns of influenza a virus in wild birds. *Science.* 2006 Apr 21;312(5772):384-8.

Olszewska E, Łaska-Mierzejewska T. Unemployment in the Polish countryside and its effect on the development and rate of maturation of rural girls. *Anthropological Review* 71(1):33-42.

Patel RB, Burke TF. Urbanization -- An Emerging Humanitarian Disaster. *N Engl J Med.* 2009; 361(8):741–43.

Salmond CE, Joseph JG, Prior IA, Stanley DG, Wessen AF. Longitudinal analysis of the relationship between blood pressure and migration: the Tokelau Island Migrant Study. *Am J Epidemiol.* 1985;122(2):291-301.

Shah SM, Loney T, Dhaheri SA, Vatanparast H, Elbarazi I, Agarwal M, Blair I, Ali R. Association between acculturation, obesity and cardiovascular risk factors among male South Asian migrants in the United Arab Emirates--a cross-sectional study. *BMC Public Health.* 2015 Feb 28;15:204. doi: 10.1186/s12889-015-1568-x.

Soares M, Müller MJ. 2017. *Type 2 diabetes in Asia: where do we go from here?.* 71:801-802.

Szklarska A, Lipowicz A, Lopuszanska M, Bielicki T, Koziel S. Biological condition of adult migrants and nonmigrants in Wrocław, Poland. *Am J Hum Biol.* 2008;20(2):139-45.

Tenkorang EY. Early onset of type 2 diabetes among visible minority and immigrant populations in Canada. *Ethn Health.* 2017 Jun; 22(3):266-284. doi: 10.1080/13557858.2016.1244623. Epub 2016 Oct 24.

Umezaki M, Ohtsuka R. Impact of rural-urban migration on fertility: a population ecology analysis in theKombio, Papua New Guinea. *J Biosoc Sci.* 1998;30(3):411-22.

Daştan İ, Erem A, Çetinkaya V. Urban and rural differences in hypertension risk factors in Turkey. *Anatol J Cardiol.* 2017 Jul;18(1):39-47. doi: 10.14744/AnatolJCardiol.2017.7452. Epub 2017 Apr 19.

Wilcove DS, Wikelski M. Going, going, gone: is animal migration disappearing. *PLoS Biol.* 2008 Jul 29;6(7):e188. doi: 10.1371/journal.pbio.0060188.

Zimmet PZ, Alberti KG, Shaw JE. 2005. Mainstreaming the metabolic syndrome: a definitive definition. *Med J Aust.* 183: 175-176.

In: Ethnicity and Syndrome X
Editors: M. Das and K. Bose
ISBN: 978-1-53618-042-8
© 2020 Nova Science Publishers, Inc.

Chapter 9

Ethnic Differences in Proinflammatory State and Syndrome X: An Overview

***Plaban Chaudhury*[1]*, Riddhi Goswami*[1]**
***and Mithun Das*[2,*]**
[1]Department of Biotechnology, Heritage Institute of Technology, Kolkata, India
[2]Department of Anthropology, Sidho-Kanho-Birsha University, Purulia, West Bengal, India

The most widely recognized of the metabolic risk factors are atherogenic dyslipidemia, elevated blood pressure, and elevated plasma glucose. Individuals with these characteristics commonly manifest a prothrombotic state and a proinflammatory state. Atherogenic dyslipidemia consists of an aggregation of lipoprotein abnormalities including elevated serum triglyceride and apolipoprotein B (apoB), increased small low density lipoprotein cholesterol (LDLc) particles, and a reduced level of high density

* Corresponding Author's Email: mithundas01@yahoo.com.

lipoprotein cholesterol (HDLc). The metabolic syndrome or syndrome X is often referred to as if it were a discrete entity with a single cause. Available data suggest that it truly is a syndrome, i.e., a grouping of atherosclerotic cardiovascular disease (ASCVD) risk factors, but one that probably has more than one cause. Regardless of cause, the syndrome identifies individuals at an elevated risk for ASCVD. The magnitude of the increased risk can vary according to which components of the syndrome are present plus the other, non-syndrome X risk factors in a particular person (Grundy et al., 2005), ethnicity and gender.

People with the syndrome X frequently have a proinflammatory state as shown by elevated cytokines (e.g., tumor necrosis factor-α, and interleukin-6) and acute-phase reactants (e.g., C-reactive protein, fibrinogen) (Pearson et al., 2003; Ridker et al., 2004). Measurement of C-reactive protein (CRP) is the simplest way to identify a proinflammatory state in clinical practice. CRP levels $\geq$ 3 mg/L can be taken to define such a state in a person without other detectable causes. If CRP is measured, the finding of an elevated level supports the need for lifestyle changes. The latter, particularly weight reduction, will reduce CRP levels and presumably will mitigate the underlying inflammatory stimulus. No drugs that act exclusively through this mechanism are available for reducing cardiovascular risk. However, several drugs used to treat other metabolic risk factors have been reported to reduce CRP levels (e.g., statins, nicotinic acid, fibrates, ACE inhibitors, and thiazolidinediones) (Jialal et al., 2001; Schieffer et al., 2004; Nesto, 2004).

Obesity is closely linked to the development of metabolic risk and also related to chronic systemic low-grade inflammation marked by altered circulating levels of adipokine and inflammatory markers (Harford et al., 2011; Bulcao et al., 2006). Thus, adipose tissue, consisting of adipocytes, immune cells and nerve/connective tissue, is now recognized as an important endocrine and metabolically active organ. The pro-inflammatory phenotype associated with excess fat mass results in low production of adiponectin and high production of leptin, CRP, interleukin-6 (IL-6) and tumor necrosis factor-α (TNF-α). Interestingly, the pro-inflammatory response appears to differ depending on body fat distribution. Because visceral adipose tissue (VAT) surrounds the internal organs and is more vascular and metabolically active than subcutaneous adipose tissue (SAT), VAT accumulation is thought to be more health hazardous—that is, increased risks of insulin resistance and related metabolic diseases—than abdominal or peripheral SAT (Hocking et al., 2013). Central adiposity differs by sex and ethnicity (Patel et al., 2013), in particular, Asian ethnicity is associated with higher VAT and African American (AA) ethnicity with lower VAT relative to whites (Conroy et al., 2011; Lim et al., 2011; Carroll et al., 2009). These variations in adipose tissue composition appear to be linked to ethnic disparities in obesity-related chronic diseases, such as higher rates of diabetes among Japanese Americans (JA) or AA at similar body mass index (BMI) levels (Maskatinec et al., 2009; Resnick et al., 1998). The hypothesis is that differences in circulating adipokines and inflammatory markers as a result of ethnic differences in the distribution of adipose tissue are partially responsible for these ethnic disparities in obesity-related disease risk (Conroy et al., 2011; Carroll et al., 2009). In a cross-sectional study, leptin, adiponectin, CRP, IL-6 and TNF-α in fasting serum samples was measured within a multiethnic population of older men and women consisting of whites, JA, Latinos, AA and Native Hawaiians (NH). Circulating levels of these biomarkers were compared across ethnic groups before and after adjustment for BMI to evaluate the plausibility of ethnic differences in biomarker levels due to differences in body fat distribution independent of weight status. It was found that older men and women with a wide range of BMI levels, ethnic differences in serum adipokine and CRP levels were detected in men and women. As compared to whites, leptin levels were lower in JA men and women and higher in AA women, adiponectin levels were lower in AA men and women and in JA and NH women, CRP was lower in JA men and women as well as in NH women and higher in AA men and women after taking into account BMI (Morimoto et al., 2014).

CRP and family history of diabetes was found to be highly associated with syndrome X in a recent study among obstetric population of Asian Indians living in and around Kolkata (*erstwhile* Calcutta), India (Goswami et al., 2019). As adiponectin is thought to play a favorable patho-physiological role in obesity-related diseases (Matsuzawa, 2010), the current evidence supports the idea that adiponectin is partially responsible for ethnic-specific disparities in obesity-related diseases (Maskarinec et al., 2009; Resnick et al., 1998). The possible relation with body fat distribution was strengthened by a study showing that variations in VAT and SAT measured by computed tomography partially explained the differences in biomarker levels across ethnic groups (Carroll et al., 2009). However, the presence of additional confounding factors was indicated by statistically significant associations for Hispanics and AA after adjustment for VAT and SAT. Therefore, ethnic differences in levels of adipokine and inflammatory marker, if they truly exist, are unlikely to be fully explained by differences in common measures of general adiposity and body fat distribution, such as BMI and waist circumference. To further elucidate the underlying mechanisms for ethnic-specific differences in biomarker levels, future studies need to examine specific fat depots or adipocyte morphology, which are not traditionally measured in epidemiologic studies, specifically, liver fat, superficial vs. deep SAT, adipocyte size or adipocyte hypertrophy and understand the important influence of genetic and lifestyle factors on adiposity (Lara-Castro et al., 2005; Mente et al., 2013; Mente et al., 201; Lara-Castro et al., 2005).

Several explanations have been proposed to explain the origin of the syndrome X. Some consider an initial insulin resistant state progressing to the other components, while others are of view that obesity is the main initiator of the syndrome (Misra et al., 2008). More recently, the chronic low-grade inflammatory condition that often accompanies the syndrome X has been implicated as a major factor both in the installation of the syndrome X and its associated patho-physiological consequences (de Ferranti & Mozaffarian, 2008). However, the inflammatory state that accompanies the syndrome X does not completely fit into the classical definition of acute or chronic inflammation, as it is not accompanied by infection; there is no massive tissue injury and the dimension of the inflammatory activation is also not large. So it is often called 'low grade' chronic inflammation or 'meta-inflammation', meaning metabolically-triggered inflammation (Hotamisligil, 2006) or even 'para-inflammation' an intermediate state between basal and inflammatory states (Medzhitov, 2008).

Whatever the term used, the inflammatory process that characterizes the syndrome X has its own unique features but its causes are far from being fully understood. Several studies support to the concept that a proinflammatory state is a component of the syndrome X because of the strong association of elevated CRP and high CRP levels impart risk for major coronary events beyond that imparted by the other metabolic risk factors. High-sensitivity CRP (hs-CRP) has been developed and used as a marker to predict coronary vascular diseases in syndrome X and it was recently used as a predictor for non-alcoholic fatty liver disease in correlation with serum markers that indicated lipid and glucose metabolism. However the reasons for a link between inflammation and syndrome X are not fully understood. One explanation may be that adipose tissue in obese persons with the syndrome X releases increased amounts of cytokines into the circulation which in turn accounts for a greater production of CRP by the liver. Another possibility is that insulin resistance per se is responsible for a higher production of cytokines. Regardless of mechanism, the finding that patients with syndrome X exhibit characteristics of a proinflammatory state provides a new and exciting connection between inflammation and metabolic processes. This connection promises to yield new insights into pathways whereby the syndrome X leads to atherosclerosis and acute coronary syndromes (Grundy, 2003). Further tissue malfunction or homeostatic imbalance of one or several physiological systems seems to be associated with inflammatory process, but it is sometimes difficult to understand how this would bring out a host defense mechanism. Instead of being beneficial, it seems to progress to a deregulated state and is implicated in the worsening of the condition. It has even been questioned whether there is any physiological counterpart for this inflammatory response. It is possible that the initial response provides short-term benefits and later on in a chronic phase it becomes maladaptive. In fact, inducible adaptive changes generally occur at the expenses of many other physiological processes and, therefore, cannot be sustained without adverse side effects caused by the decline in the affected functions (Medzhitov, 2008). It is difficult to pin point a single cause for the activation of inflammation, as it is a sequential events related to the deterioration of metabolic homeostasis. Apparently, metabolic overload evokes several stress reactions including oxidative, inflammatory, organelle and cell hypertrophy stresses, generating vicious cycles that amplify each other leading to dysfunction (Monteiro &Azevedo, 2010). The difficulty in the management of the syndrome is linked to its multi-factorial nature where environmental, genetic and psychosocial factors may play a vital role. Undoubtedly, the connections between inflammation and metabolism are complex and present a challenge for new research. The awareness of the importance of inflammation in the syndrome X may help to develop new strategies for the prevention and treatment of syndrome X related disorders (Sharma, 2011).

Hence, proinflammatory state should seriously be taken in to consideration for proper screening and management of syndrome X across ethnicity and gender.

REFERENCES

Bulcao C, Ferreira SR, Giuffrida FM, Ribeiro-Filho FF. The new adipose tissue and adipocytokines. *Curr Diabetes Rev.* 2006; 2: 19–28.

Carroll JF, Fulda KG, Chiapa AL, Rodriquez M, Phelps DR, Cardarelli KM et al. Impact of race/ethnicity on the relationship between visceral fat and inflammatory biomarkers. *Obesity (Silver Spring).* 2009; 17: 1420–1427.

Conroy SM, Chai W, Lim U, Franke AA, Cooney RV, Maskarinec G. Leptin, Adiponectin,and Obesity among Caucasian and Asian Women. *Mediators Inflamm.* 2011: 253580.

de Ferranti S, Mozaffarian D. The perfect storm: obesity, adipocyte dysfunction, and metabolic consequences. *Clin Chem.* 2008; 54: 945–55.

Fantuzzi G. Adipose tissue, adipokines, and inflammation. *J Allergy ClinImmunol.* 2005; 115: 911–919.

Fujimoto WY. The importance of insulin resistance in the pathogenesis of type 2 diabetes mellitus. *Am J Med.* 2000; 108: 9S–14S.

Geer EB, Shen W. Gender differences in insulin resistance, body composition, and energy balance. *Gend Med.* 2009; 6: 60–75.

Goswami R, Das M, Lodh I. C-reactive protein and family history: a future threat towards diabetes and syndrome X. In *Obesity and Syndrome X* ed. Das & Bose. 2019. 201-2014.

Grundy SM, Cleeman JI, Daniels SR, et al. Diagnosis and Management of the Metabolic Syndrome. *Circulation.* 2005; 112: 2735-2752

Grundy SM. Inflammation, metabolic syndrome, and dietresponsiveness. *Circulation*. 2003; 108: 126–128.

Harford KA, Reynolds CM, Mc Gillicuddy FC, Roche HM. Fats inflammation and insulin resistance: insights to the role of macrophage and T-cell accumulation in adipose tissue. *Proc Nutr Soc*. 2011; 70: 408–417.

Hocking S, Samocha-Bonet D, Milner KL, Greenfield JR, Chisholm DJ. Adiposity and Insulin Resistance in Humans: The Role of the Different Tissue and Cellular Lipid Depots. *Endocr Rev*. 2013; 34: 463–500.

Hotamisligil GS. Inflammation and metabolic disorders. *Nature*. 2006; 444: 860–867.

Jialal I, Stein D, Balis D, Grundy SM, Adams-Huet B, Devaraj S. Effect of hydroxyl methyl glutaryl coenzyme a reductase inhibitor therapy on high sensitive C-reactive protein levels. *Circulation*. 2001; 103:b1933–1935.

Lara-Castro C, Hunter GR, Lovejoy JC, Gower BA, Fernandez JR. Association of the intestinal fatty acid-binding protein Ala54Thr polymorphism and abdominal adipose tissue in African-American and Caucasian women. *J Clin Endocrinol Metab.* 2005; 90: 1196–1201.

Lara-Castro C, Hunter GR, Lovejoy JC, Gower BA, Fernandez JR. Apolipoprotein A-II polymorphism and visceral adiposity in African-American and white women. *Obes Res*. 2005; 13: 507–512.

Lim U, Ernst T, Buchthal SD, Latch M, Albright CL, Wilkens LR et al. Asian women have greater abdominal and visceral adiposity than Caucasian women with similar body mass index. *Nutr Diabetes*. 2011; 1: e6.

Maskarinec G, Erber E, Grandinetti A, Verheus M, Oum R, Hopping BN et al. Diabetes incidence based on linkages with health plans: the multiethnic cohort. *Diabetes*. 2009; 58: 1732–1738.

Matsuzawa Y. Adiponectin: a key player in obesity related disorders. *Curr Pharm Des*. 2010; 16: 1896–1901.

Medzhitov R. Origin and physiological roles of inflammation. *Nature*. 2008; 454: 428–35.

Mente A, Meyre D, Lanktree MB, Heydarpour M, Davis AD, Miller R et al. Causal Relationship between Adiponectin and Metabolic Traits: A Mendelian Randomization Study in a Multiethnic Population. *PLoS One*. 2013; 8: e66808.

Mente A, Razak F, Blankenberg S, Vuksan V, Davis AD, Miller R et al. Ethnic variation in adiponectin and leptin levels and their association with adiposity and insulin resistance. *Diabetes Care*. 2010; 33: 1629–1634.

Mittra S, Bansal VS, Bhatnagar PK. From a glucocentric to alipocentric approach towards metabolic syndrome. *Drug Discov Today*. 2008; 13: 211–8.

Monteiro R, Azevedo I. Chronic inflammation in obesity and the metabolic syndrome. *Mediat Inflamm*. 2010; Article ID 289645. doi: 10.1155/ 2010/289645.

Nesto R. C-reactive protein, its role in inflammation, Type 2 diabetes and cardiovascular disease, and the effects of insulin-sensitizing treatment with thiazolidinediones. *Diabet Med*. 2004; 21: 810–817.

Patel PS, Buras ED, Balasubramanyam A. The role of the immune system in obesity and insulin resistance. *J Obes* 2013; 2013: 616193.

Pearson TA, Mensah GA, Alexander RW, Anderson JL, Cannon RO III,Criqui M, Fadl YY, Fortmann SP, Hong Y, Myers GL, Rifai N, Smith SC Jr, Taubert K, Tracy RP, Vinicor F; Centers for Disease Control and Prevention; American Heart Association. Markers of inflammation and cardiovascular disease: application to clinical and public health practice: a statement for healthcare professionals from the Centers for Disease Control and Prevention and the American Heart Association. *Circulation*. 2003; 107: 499 –511.

Resnick HE, Valsania P, Halter JB, Lin X. Differential effects of BMI on diabetes risk among black and white Americans. *Diabetes Care*. 1998; 21: 1828–1835.

Ridker PM, Buring JE, Cook NR, Rifai N. C-reactive protein, the metabolic syndrome, and the risk of incident cardiovascular events: an8-year follow-up of 14 719 initially healthy American women. *Circulation*. 2003; 107: 391–397.

Ridker PM, Wilson PW, Grundy SM. Should C-reactive protein be added to metabolic syndrome and to assessment of global cardiovascular risk? *Circulation*. 2004; 109: 2818 –2825.

Rose DP, Haffner SM, Baillargeon J. Adiposity, the metabolic syndrome, and breast cancer in African-American and white American women. *Endocr Rev*. 2007; 28: 763–777.

Schieffer B, Bunte C, Witte J, Hoeper K, Boger RH, Schwedhelm E, Drexler H. Comparative effects of AT1-antagonism and angiotensin converting enzyme inhibition on markers of inflammation and platelet aggregation in patients with coronary artery disease. *J Am Coll Cardiol*. 2004; 44: 362–368.

Sharma Praveen, Inflammation and the Metabolic Syndrome. *Indian J Clin Biochem*. 2011; 26: 317-318.

Yehuda-Shnaidman E, Schwartz B. Mechanisms linking obesity, inflammation and altered metabolism to colon carcinogenesis. *Obes Rev* 2012; 13: 1083–1095.

In: Ethnicity and Syndrome X
Editors: M. Das and K. Bose
ISBN: 978-1-53618-042-8
© 2020 Nova Science Publishers, Inc.

Chapter 10

ANTHROPOMETRIC MEASURES, BODY COMPOSITION AND THE RISK OF HYPERTENSION: A STUDY ON INDIAN TRIBES

Gautam Kumar Kshatriya* and Anjali Kumari
Department of Anthropology, University of Delhi, Delhi, India

INTRODUCTION

High blood pressure is the leading cause of global health risk in the World that accounts 13% of deaths globally. Hypertension is considered as one of the key risk factors that lead to heart attack, stroke, kidney failure, premature death and disability (WHO, 2014). It is reported that elevated blood pressure is a "third killer" disease accounting for 1 in every 8 deaths worldwide (WHO, 2013). Changing lifestyle, sedentary behavior and modernization played a significant role in increasing the prevalence of

* Corresponding Author's Email: g26_51@yahoo.co.in.

hypertension (WHO, 2010; 2014). Various factors were identified as a major risk for predicting increased blood pressure such as obesity, body fat percentage and abdominal obesity: [minimum waist circumference (MWC)], waist circumference based indices - waist hip ratio (WHR), waist height ratio (WHtR), body mass index (BMI) (Bose et al., 2003; Shanthirani et al., 2003; Ghosh, 2007; Sarkar et al., 2009; Mungreiphy et al., 2011, Dua et al., 2014; Laxmaiah et al., 2015; Gupta, 2016; Kshatriya & Acharya, 2016). BMI was found as the most traditional method for defining overweight and obesity which indicate overall obesity and hence, it cannot be used to reflect abdominal obesity (WHO, 2008; Huxley et al., 2010). Various studies have reported MWC, WHR, WHtR, visceral fat (VF), subcutaneous fat and body fat percentage as better indicators of abdominal obesity as compared to BMI (WHO, 1998; Yusuf et al., 2014; Seidell, 2010). Hypertension is alarmingly increasing in both developed and developing countries especially in poor and vulnerable groups of population. Many studies have reported the prevalence of hypertension worldwide (Hajjar et al., 2006; Lacruz et al., 2015; Mills et al., 2016; Divney et al., 2018; Sanuade et al., 2018). Similarly, in Indian context, prevalence of hypertension have been reported among various populations of different ethnicities (Ghosh, 2007; Kshatriya & Acharya, 2016; Das et al., 2010; Anchala et al., 2014; Midha et al., Gupta et al., 2012). Indian tribal population also experienced serious health issues of hypertension (Kshatriya & Acharya, 2016; NIN, 2009; Manimunda et al., 2011; Meshram et al., 2012; Rizwan et al., 2014; Kshatriya & Acharya, 2019). But in terms of coverage, sample size; few studies were conducted so far in context of tribal communities. The present study gives an insight on the health status of the selected nine tribes living in varied environmental settings and practicing different cultures. This work can be beneficial for planning similar studies and interventions among other population groups across India.

The present study attempts to find out the association of anthropometric measures and body composition with the risk of hypertension among Indian tribes.

Materials and Methods

Area and People

The present study included nine major tribes namely Santal, Bhumij and Bathudi from Mayurbhanj district of Odisha, and Kora, Oraon and Santal from Birbhum district of West Bengal and Kukna, Dhodia and Chaudhury from Valsad district of Gujarat as shown in Figure 1. The study was conducted in selected tribal villages on the basis of their population concentration.

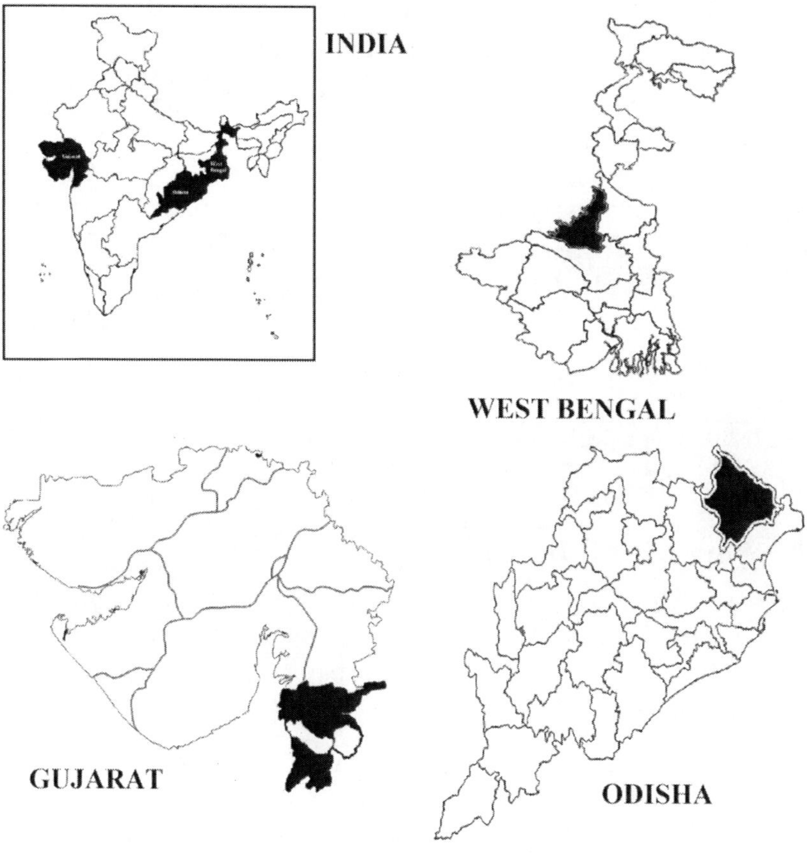

Figure 1. Map of India highlighting selected states of the fieldwork.

Sampling and Study Design

Data collection was based on a simple random sampling method. During January 2011 to December 2013, we conducted a cross-sectional study among 1066 adult males and 1090 females constituting a total of 2156 adult participants aged 20-60 years. Simple random sampling method was used in each study areas. The response rate for the study was 80% and a total sample size of 2156 was used in the present study.

Table 1 shows the absolute number of males and females of each tribal groups of the present study.

Table1. Absolute number of males and females for each tribal group (N = 2156)

Name of tribes	Males (n = 1066)	Females (n = 1090)
Bathudi	119	121
Bhumij	116	122
Chaudhari	120	121
Dhodia	121	120
Kora	114	121
Kukna	120	120
Oraon	112	124
Santal (O)	121	119
Santal WB	123	122

O-Odisha; WB-West Bengal.

Anthropometric Measurements

A standard questionnaire was used to collect data on characteristics such as ethnicity, age and sex of the participants. Standard techniques were followed while taking all the anthropometric measurements such as height, minimum waist circumference (MWC), mid upper arm circumference (MUAC), maximum hip circumference and sum of four skinfolds (SF4) as mentioned by Lohman et al., (1988). The standing height and weight were measured to the nearest of 0.1 cm and 0.1 kg respectively. A movable anthropometer was used to measure the height.

BMI was calculated as weight in kilogram (kg) divided by height in meter squared (kg/m^2). WHtR was calculated by dividing waist circumference to height and WHR was calculated as the ratio of waist circumference to hip circumference. Skinfold thickness at biceps, triceps, subscapular and suprailiac were taken using Holtain skinfold caliper and sum of these four skinfolds (SF4) was used for defining obesity in the present study.

Body Composition Measures

Measures such as body fat percentage (PBF) and visceral fat (VF) were collected using the Omron Karada Scan Body Composition Monitor (Omron Health Care Co., Kyoto, Japan, 2008). Participants were requested to come with light clothes prior to the measurement.

Blood Pressure

A standard procedure of American Heart Association guidelines was followed for measuring the blood pressure (Liz, 2005). Participants with blood pressure $\geq$140/90 mmHg were considered as hypertensive (Choanian, 2003).

Exclusion Criteria

Those participants who were not willing to participate were excluded from the study. Participants with severe chronic diseases during the past one year were also excluded from the study.

Statistical Analysis

Data were analyzed using SPSS version 16.0 for Windows (SPSS Inc., Chicago, Illinois, USA). Descriptive statistics such as mean and standard deviation (SD) were used for selected anthropometric measurements and blood pressure variables such as SBP (systolic blood pressure) and DBP (diastolic blood pressure) to describe the characteristics of the studied populations. Principal component analysis (PCA) is used to group the quantitatively measured variables into components. In the present study, PCA was used to understand the underlying causal factors that explained most of the variance in the selected population for predicting hypertension. The particular variables used in the PCA were MWC, MUAC, BMI, WHR, WHtR, SF4, VF and PBF and high blood pressure (≥140/90 mmHg) was used as selection variables in the SPSS. Varimax rotation is an orthogonal rotation in which the factors are assumed to act independently (maximum likelihood), and was used in this study (Comrey& Lee, 2013). Variables in the two components with component loading coefficients ≥0.4 were used for further interpretation (Comrey& Lee, 2013; Long, 1983; Stevens, 2012, Hodge et al., 2001). The Eigen value (>1) of the two components were generated to estimate the factor variances.

RESULTS

Table 2 shows the characteristics of the studied nine tribal populations from Odisha, West Bengal and Gujarat. All the selected variables like anthropometric measures (minimum waist circumference-MWC, mid upper arm circumference- MUAC and sum of four skinfolds- SF4), adiposity indices (body mass index-BMI, waist hip ratio-WHR and waist height ratio-WHtR) and body composition (weight, PBF and VF) were found to be statistically significant at $p < 0.001$. Variables like MWC, MUAC, BMI, WHR, WHtR, SF4 and VF showed higher mean difference among adult males as compared to females whereas age, PBF, SBP and DBP were found higher in females in comparison to males.

Table 2. Characteristics of the studied tribal populations (N = 2156)

Tribe	Sex		Age	MWC	SBP	DBP	PBF	VF	BMI	WHR	WHtR	SF4	MUAC
Bathudi	M	Mean	39.97	74.77	125.44	75.79	16.61	4.11	19.46	0.92	0.48	36.34	25.55
		SD	±12.46	±7.66	±17.94	±11.64	±5.39	±3.00	±2.67	±0.05	±0.05	±15.29	±2.28
	F	Mean	40.17	66.53	132.75	86.23	24.34	2.18	17.97	0.84	0.45	34.67	21.39
		SD	±12.20	±4.56	±23.21	±14.67	±6.09	±1.54	±2.76	±0.05	±0.04	±12.92	±2.35
Bhumij	M	Mean	42.22	77.69	128.74	76.42	18.95	5.84	20.93	0.90	0.48	42.60	25.17
		SD	±12.52	±8.91	±21.40	±13.25	±6.20	±3.39	±3.05	±0.05	±0.05	±28.17	±6.46
	F	Mean	40.83	68.91	129.94	82.89	27.25	3.07	19.70	0.84	0.46	37.80	22.33
		SD	±11.43	±5.96	±25.14	±13.20	±5.81	±2.28	±2.94	±0.05	±0.04	±13.24	±2.29
Kora	M	Mean	40.05	68.27	124.91	80.32	17.29	3.53	18.94	0.86	0.43	24.22	22.80
		SD	±12.86	±6.26	±21.00	±11.50	±6.48	±2.04	±1.97	±0.06	±0.04	±6.60	±1.77
	F	Mean	40.16	61.87	124.51	79.26	23.51	2.07	17.64	0.82	0.42	29.65	21.04
		SD	±12.32	±5.60	±22.31	±14.08	±6.54	±1.34	±2.86	±0.06	±0.04	±11.30	±3.57
Oraon	M	Mean	39.04	70.71	124.10	79.63	17.20	4.21	19.58	0.86	0.44	28.38	24.03
		SD	±12.60	±6.68	±15.41	±9.93	±6.51	±2.69	±2.51	±0.05	±0.04	±10.00	±2.22
	F	Mean	39.74	63.11	130.90	84.68	25.38	2.21	18.13	0.81	0.43	27.94	21.19
		SD	±11.79	±6.06	±20.00	±13.98	±6.07	±1.74	±2.79	±0.05	±0.04	±10.94	±1.97
Santal (O)	M	Mean	41.38	75.25	125.79	76.09	18.73	4.89	20.20	0.91	0.47	31.60	25.97
		SD	±13.37	±8.02	±16.89	±13.10	±6.24	±2.99	±2.80	±0.06	±0.05	±12.63	±5.69
	F	Mean	39.25	71.14	125.42	82.21	27.72	3.50	20.30	0.85	0.48	46.64	23.22
		SD	±12.57	±7.81	±15.07	±10.60	±7.02	±2.69	±3.04	±0.06	±0.05	±20.54	±2.53
Santal WB	M	Mean	39.81	71.67	127.54	79.65	18.43	4.50	19.88	0.87	0.44	28.38	23.60
		SD	±13.29	±7.70	±18.22	±11.05	±5.71	±2.83	±2.59	±0.06	±0.05	±10.93	±2.20
	F	Mean	39.76	66.14	123.93	78.60	27.29	3.05	19.46	0.82	0.44	37.67	22.19
		SD	±12.13	±6.28	±23.96	±13.22	±6.09	±2.39	±3.19	±0.05	±0.04	±14.57	±2.25
Dhodia	M	Mean	41.55	79.48	129.04	80.16	23.18	5.74	20.52	0.94	0.49	32.15	25.91
		SD	±11.62	±10.86	±20.43	±11.54	±5.77	±3.71	±3.20	±0.07	±0.06	±16.3	±2.75
	F	Mean	40.38	69.25	129.57	82.26	31.36	4.02	20.68	0.82	0.46	48.5	23.12
		SD	±11.63	±8.57	±20.37	±13.5	±5.92	±2.89	±3.45	±0.05	±0.05	±18.65	±2.52
Kukna	M	Mean	40.09	78.87	128.35	79.34	21.70	5.19	20.30	0.94	0.48	33.62	26.28
		SD	±12.38	±9.96	±17.40	±11.09	±6.67	±3.42	±3.13	±0.06	±0.05	±14.59	±2.80
	F	Mean	40.05	68.28	127.17	80.12	30.09	3.28	19.84	0.82	0.46	46.54	22.94
		SD	±11.64	±7.50	±16.75	±9.52	±5.69	±2.12	±2.79	±0.05	±0.05	±14.74	±2.34
Chaudhari	M	Mean	40.87	78.26	125.69	75.14	22.09	5.11	19.81	0.95	0.48	29.20	25.56
		SD	±13.18	±10.64	±23.44	±11.53	±5.69	±4.46	±3.11	±0.07	±0.06	±11.70	±2.49
	F	Mean	40.47	64.15	123.71	80.12	28.18	2.79	18.91	0.78	0.42	41.63	21.88
		SD	±11.63	±7.48	±21.65	±13.79	±6.07	±1.91	±2.91	±0.05	±0.05	±27.26	±2.20

MWC- minimum waist circumference; MUAC- mid-upper circumference; VF- visceral fat; BMI-body mass index; WHR-waist hip ratio; WHtR- waist height ratio.

SF4- sum of four skinfolds; PBF- body fat percentage; SBP-systolic blood pressure; DBP-diastolic blood pressure.

Table 3. Age and sex wise prevalence of hypertension in each selected tribe of India

Name of the tribes	Males (n = 1066)				Females (n = 1090)			
	20-30	31-40	41-50	51-60	20-30	31-40	41-50	51-60
Bathudi	0	3.1	3.7	13.3	3.2	13.3	43.3	16.7
Bhumij	3.6	14.3	17.2	16.1	9.4	6.7	20	30
Chaudhuri	3.2	3.4	0	6.7	0	3.3	12.9	20
Dhodia	3.3	9.4	15.2	23.1	6.7	6.7	23.3	20
Kora	0	0	11.1	17.9	0	9.7	16.7	30
Kukna	6.2	13.3	21.4	13.3	3.3	0	10	23.3
Oraon	3.4	6.7	13.3	13	3	16.7	40	35.5
Santal (O)	0	6.7	13.6	21.1	3.2	7.1	20	3.3
Santal (WB)	3	6.7	10	20	0	0	16.7	40

Table 3 shows age and sex- wise prevalence of hypertension in each selected tribes of India. In males, the percentage of hypertension was found to be increased in Bathudi, Chaudhuri, Dhodia, Kora, Santal of Odisha (O) and Santal of West Bengal (WB) among all the age groups. Similar results were found in females of Bhumij, Chaudhuri, Kora, Kukna and Santal of WB. On the other hand, in males, the percentage of high blood pressure was found to be slightly decreased in the age groups ranged from 41 to 50 years and 51 to 60 years. Similar findings were found in females of Bathudi, Dhodia, Oraon and Santal of Odisha (O).

Table 4 (a) shows factor loadings of principal component analysis. Principal component analysis (PCA) identified two components as component 1(PC1) and component 2 (PC2). PC1 was found with high loading variables like, MWC (0.96), MUAC (0.79), BMI (0.78), WHR (0.86), WHtR (0.90), SF4 (0.54)) and VF (0.86). The variance explained in PC1 was 59.7% of total variance observed for high blood pressure. Similarly, PC2 was found with high loading variables like, BMI (0.47), SF4 (0.68) and PBF (0.88). The cumulative variance was 81.1% of the total variance observed for high blood pressure. SF4 was found as an overlapping variable in both components (PC1 and PC2). In males, PC 1 [MUAC (0.68), MWC (0.95), BMI (0.89), WHR (0.82), WHtR (0.95), SF4 (0.83), PBF (0.50) and VF (0.92) revealed 69.2% of variance, while in females PC 1

[MUAC (0.82), MWC (0.67), BMI (0.93), WHtR (0.61), SF4 (0.82), PBF (0.71) and VF (0.93)] revealed 59.4% of variance observed for high blood pressure respectively. In females, PC 2 [MWC (0.68), WHR (0.96) and WHtR (0.74)] revealed 27.2% of variance observed for high blood pressure.

Table 4 (b) represents logistic regression analysis that was performed to ascertain the effects of PC scores 1 and PC scores 2 on the likelihood that participants have hypertension. In the present Table 4, PC 1 shows 1.23 times and PC 2 shows 1.40 times more likely to cause hypertension in the studied tribal populations of India. On the other hand, males exhibit 2.01 times more likely to have hypertension due to PC 1, while females show 1.20 times more likely to have hypertension due to PC 2. It is remarkably observed that PC 1 [$p < 0.01$, 95% C.I (1.06-1.43)] and PC 2 [$p < 0.001$, 95% C.I (1.25-1.57)] were found as the significant predictors of high blood pressure in the total studied population. In case of males, PC 1 [$p < 0.001$, 95% C.I (1.58-2.56)], while in females PC 2 [$p < 0.05$, 95% C.I (0.99-1.45)] were found as significant predictors of hypertension.

Table 4 (a). Component loadings of the principal components among studied tribes of India

	Total Populations (N = 2156)		Females (n-1090)		Males (n = 1060)
Variables	PC 1	PC 2	PC 1	PC 2	PC 1
MWC (cm)	0.96	0.08	0.67	0.68	0.95
MUAC (cm)	0.79	0.16	0.82	0.28	0.68
BMI (kg/m2)	0.78	0.47	0.93	0.16	0.89
WHR	0.86	-0.27	0.001	0.96	0.82
WHtR	0.90	0.23	0.61	0.74	0.95
SF4 (mm)	0.54	0.68	0.82	0.28	0.83
VF (%)	0.86	0.28	0.93	0.10	0.92
PBF	-0.058	0.88	0.71	0.16	0.50
Variance%	59.71	21.4	54.94	27.24	69.20
Cumulative variance%	-	81.10	-	82.18	-
Eigen values	5.13	1.35	5.34	1.22	5.53

MWC- minimum waist circumference; MUAC- mid upper arm circumference; BMI-body mass index; WHR- waist hip ratio; WHtR- waist height ratio.

SF4- sum of four skinfolds; VF- visceral fat and PBF- Percent body fat loading value ≥0.4.

Table 4 (b). Logistic regression analysis using PCA scores for high blood pressure (N = 2156)

High blood pressure (≥140/90 mm Hg)	Standardized coefficients (β)	S.E	Exp (β)	p-value	95% C.I
Total Population					
PC score 1	0.21	0.07	1.23	0.005	1.06-1.43
PC score 2	0.33	0.05	1.40	0.001	1.25-1.57
Males					
PC score 1	0.70	0.12	2.01	0.001	1.58-2.56
Females					
PC score 1	0.18	0.16	1.19	0.26	0.87-1.64
PC score 2	0.19	0.09	1.20	0.05	0.99-1.45

PCA- Principal component analysis; PC- Principal components.

DISCUSSION

The present study attempts to find out the associations of anthropometric measures and body composition with the risk of hypertension among Indian tribes. The present findings showed two components with high component loadings where PC1 (MUAC, MWC, BMI, WHR, WHtR, SF4 and VF) explained 59.7% of the variance observed for high blood pressure in the total population. Similarly, PC2 shows high component loadings where three selected variables (BMI, SF4 and PBF) explained 21.7% of the variance observed for high blood pressure. It was remarkably observed that PC 1 was found to be overlapping components indicating the risk of hypertension in the total, males and females of the studied tribes. Logistic regression analysis (LRA) shows that these two components predict high blood pressure in the selected tribal groups of India. In LRA, PC 1 ($p < 0.01$) and PC 2 ($p < 0.001$) showed highly significant predictor of hypertension in the total populations. On the other hand, in males, PC 1 ($p < 0.001$) while PC 2 ($p < 0.05$) in case of females showed significant predictor of hypertension in the studied tribes.

In the present study the prevalence of hypertension was found slightly higher in females than males in each selected tribes of India. The prevalence of hypertension was observed to be increasing with increase in age in both the sexes in the young and middle adults in the present study. Similar findings were reported by Reddy et al., (2006) and Gupta et al., (2012), while a slight fluctuation was also found in the age groups of 41-60 years in the present study. Reddy et al., (2015) reported 7.2% of prevalence of hypertension among young adults aged 18-25 years. Shakya et al., (2012) also reported high prevalence of hypertension among young adults of Nepal. This shows that lifestyle diseases not only affecting elder generation of India but also the young adults of Indian populations (Chakma et al., 2017).

Anthropometric measures such as MWC, WHR, WHtR, VF and PBF has been used as the adiposity markers with strong association to hypertension in the worldwide studies (Fox et al., 2007; Zhou et al., 2009; Browning et al., 2010; Li et al., 2013). Various studies have been reporting the adverse impact of body fat on blood pressure (Midha et al., 2014; Gupta et al., 2012; Rizwan et al., 2014; Aggarwal et al., 2012) MWC and MWC based indices like WHR and WHtR are considered as a useful indicator for understanding the distribution of body fat in comparison to BMI (WHO, 2008; Huxley et al., 2010; Seidell, 2010). These indices were indicators of abdominal obesity and thereby played significant role in predicting hypertension risk (Kshatriya & Acharya, 2016, Kshatriya & Acharya, 2019; Almeida et al., 2016; Taing et al., 2016). Studies reported that PBF could accurately reflect body composition than BMI (Bandyopadhyay, 2007; Imamura et al., 2008). Correspondingly, PBF and VF were found to be strongly associated with hypertension and prehypertension (Fox et al., 2007, Hayashi et al., 2004; Jiang et al., 2016). In addition, to these measures, other variables like MUAC, VF, SF4 and PBF indicates body fat distribution predicting risk of hypertension in the present study. The findings of the present study revealed that internal fat deposition, regional and overall obesity all together have a great impact in increasing the risk of hypertension. Consequently, we could use it further to make it more valid and reliable. The present study covers considerable number of sample size to report hypertension risk factors among nine selected Indian tribes. Further, applications of anthropometry and body composition played a significant role in determining the hypertension risk. Henceforth, through this easy, inexpensive and reliable approach, we can study more populations in low resource settings in other parts of India.

Limitation of the Study

The present study do not represent the diverse Indian tribal populations landscape, therefore more studies need to be done for better understanding of the hypertension trends observed in Indian tribes. Incorporation of blood sample would have provided us a better understanding of their metabolic health conditions.

CONCLUSION

The present finding shows MWC, WHR, WHtR, VF and PBF as significant predictors for determining hypertension risk in Indian tribes. Central obesity and internal fat deposition could alter the physiological and metabolic activity of the body and therefore, causing a detrimental change in health status of the tribal groups of India. A follow-up study need to be done to aware the people about the hypertension cause, risk and its severe health consequences through academicians, researchers, scientists, policy makers and other governmental and non-governmental organizations. This work can be beneficial for planning similar studies and interventions among other population groups across India.

ACKNOWLEDGMENTS

The help rendered by Prof. Satwanti Kapoor, University of Delhi and Dr Arnab Ghosh, Visva Bharati, Santiniketan in the formulation of the research problem is greatly appreciated. We express our gratitude to Mr. Subhendu Kumar Acharya, Miss Hemlata and Mr Gajanan for participating in the data collection. We sincerely acknowledge the support and co-operation of the participants of the selected villages.

Funding

This study was funded to GKK by the Indian Council of Medical Research (ICMR), Government of India, bearing project reference number [5/4/8-2/2010 NCD II].

Conflict of Interest

The authors declare that there is no conflict of interest.

REFERENCES

Aggarwal P., Jadeja J. M., Nair G. B., et al., Relationship of anthropometric adiposity indices with blood pressure in urban community of Ahmedabad. *The Southeast Asian Journal of Case Report and Review*. 2012. 1(1), 29-29.

Almeida J. B., Kian K. O., Lima R. C., et al., Total and abdominal adiposity and hypertension in indigenous women in Midwest Brazil. *PloS one*. 2016 Jun 13; 11(6):e0155528.

Anchala R., Kannuri N. K., Pant H., et al., Hypertension in India: a systematic review and meta-analysis of prevalence, awareness, and control of hypertension. *Journal of Hypertension*. 2014 Jun; 32(6):1170.

Bandyopadhyay A. Anthropometry and body composition in soccer and volleyball players in West Bengal, India. *Journal of Physiological Anthropology*. 2007; 26(4):501-5.

Bose K., Ghosh A., Roy S., Gangopadhyay S. Blood pressure and waist circumference: an empirical study of the effects of waist circumference on blood pressure among Bengaleemale jute mill workers of Belur, West Bengal, India. *Journal of Physiological Anthropology and Applied Human Science*. 2003; 22(4):169-73.

Browning L. M., Hsieh S. D., Ashwell M. A systematic review of waist-to-height ratio as a screening tool for the prediction of cardiovascular disease and diabetes: 0·5 could be a suitable global boundary value. *Nutrition research reviews*. 2010 Dec; 23(2):247-69.

Chakma T., Kavishwar A., Sharma R. K., et al., High prevalence of hypertension and its selected risk factors among adult tribal population in Central India. *Pathogens and Global Health*. 2017 Oct 3; 111(7):343-50.

Chobanian A. V. National heart, lung, and blood institute joint national committee on prevention, detection, evaluation, and treatment of high blood pressure; national high blood pressure education program coordinating committee: the seventh report of the joint national committee on prevention, detection, evaluation, and treatment of high blood pressure: the JNC 7 report. *JAMA*. 2003; 289: 2560-72.

Comrey A. L., Lee H. B. A first course in factor analysis. *Psychology press;* 2013 Nov 12.

Das M., Pal S., Ghosh A. Factor analysis of risk variables associated with metabolic syndrome in adult Asian Indians. *Journal of cardiovascular disease research*. 2010 Apr 1; 1(2):86-91.

Divney A. A., Echeverria S. E., Thorpe L. E., et al., Hypertension prevalence jointly influenced by acculturation and gender in US immigrant groups. *American journal of hypertension*. 2018 Aug 25; 32(1):104-11.

Dua S., Bhuker M., Sharma P., et al., Body mass index relates to blood pressure among adults. *North American journal of medical sciences*. 2014 Feb; 6(2):89.

Fox C. S., Massaro J. M., Hoffmann U., et al., Abdominal visceral and subcutaneous adipose tissue compartments. *Circulation*. 2007; 116: 39e48.

Ghosh A. Factor analysis of risk variables associated with metabolic syndrome in Asian Indian adolescents. *Am J Hum Biol. 2007*; 19:34e40.

Gupta M., Parashar P., Nath B., et al., An epidemiological study on hypertension and its dietary correlates in a rural population of Meerut. *Indian Journal of Community Health*. 2012 Jun 30; 24(2):161-5.

Gupta R. Convergence in urban-rural prevalence of hypertension in India. *Journal of Human Hypertension*. 2016 Feb; 30(2):79.

Hajjar I., Kotchen J. M., Kotchen T. A. Hypertension: trends in prevalence, incidence, and control. *Annu. Rev. Public Health*. 2006 Apr 21; 27:465-90.

Hayashi T., Boyko E. J., Leonetti D. L., et al., Visceral adiposity is an independent predictor of incident hypertension in Japanese Americans. *Annals of internal medicine*. 2004 Jun 15; 140(12):992.

Hodge A. M., Boyko E. J., de Courten M., et al., Leptin and other components of the Metabolic Syndrome in Mauritius - a factor analysis. *International journal of obesity*. 2001 Jan; 25(1):126.

Huxley R., Mendis S., Zheleznyakov E., et al., Body mass index, waist circumference and waist: hip ratio as predictors of cardiovascular ris - a review of the literature. *European journal of clinical nutrition*. 2010 Jan; 64(1):16.

Imamura Y., Uto H., Oketani M., et al., Association between changes in body composition and the increasing prevalence of fatty liver in Japanese men. *Hepatology Research*. 2008 Nov; 38(11):1083-6.

Jiang J., Deng S., Chen Y., et al., Comparison of visceral and body fat indices and anthropometric measures in relation to untreated hypertension by age and gender among Chinese. *International journal of cardiology*. 2016 Sep 15; 219:204-11.

Kshatriya G. K., Acharya S. K. Triple burden of obesity, undernutrition, and cardiovascular disease risk among Indian tribes. *PloS one*. 2016 Jan 25; 11(1):e0147934.

Kshatriya G., Kumari, Acharya. Comparing the ability of anthropometric indicator in determining the prevalence of hypertension among Indian tribes. *Diabetes & Metabolic Syndrome: Clinical Research & Reviews*. 2019. 13 (2019): 696-706.

Lacruz M. E., Kluttig A., Hartwig S., et al., Prevalence and incidence of hypertension in the general adult population: results of the CARLA-cohort study. *Medicine*. 2015 Jun; 94(22).

Laxmaiah A., Meshram I. I., Arlappa N., et al., Socio-economic & demographic determinants of hypertension & knowledge, practices &

risk behaviour of tribals in India. *The Indian Journal of medical research.* 2015 May; 141(5):697.

Li W. C., Chen I. C., Chang Y. C., et al., Waist-to-height ratio, waist circumference, and body mass index as indices of cardiometabolic risk among 36,642 Taiwanese adults. *European journal of nutrition.* 2013 Feb 1; 52(1):57-65.

Liz S. New AHA recommendations for blood pressure measurement: American heart association practice guidelines. *Am Fam Physician.* 2005; 72(7):1391-8.

Lohman T. G., Roche A. F., Martorell R. *Anthropometric Standardization Reference Manual.* Chicago: Human Kinetics Books. 1988.

Long J. S. *Confirmatory factor analysis: A preface to LISREL.* Sage Publications; 1983 Sep 1.

Manimunda S. P., Sugunan A. P., Benegal V., et al., Association of hypertension with risk factors & hypertension related behaviour among the aboriginal Nicobarese tribe living in Car Nicobar Island, India. *The Indian journal of medical research.* 2011 Mar; 133(3):287.

Meshram I. I., Arlappa N., Balkrishna N., et al., Prevalence of hypertension, its correlates and awareness among adult tribal population of Kerala state, India. *Journal of postgraduate medici*ne. 2012 Oct 1; 58(4):255.

Midha T., Krishna V., Nath B., et al., Cut-off of body mass index and waist circumference to predict hypertension in Indian adults. *World Journal of Clinical Cases: WJCC.* 2014 Jul 16; 2(7):272.

Mills K. T., Bundy J. D., Kelly T. N., et al., Global disparities of hypertension prevalence and control: a systematic analysis of population-based studies from 90 countries. *Circulation.* 2016 Aug 9; 134(6):441-50.

Mungreiphy N. K., Kapoor S., Sinha R. Association between BMI, blood pressure, and age: study among Tangkhul Naga tribal males of Northeast India. *Journal of Anthropology.* 2011 Dec 25; 2011.

National Nutrition Monitoring Bureau. Diet and Nutritional Status of Tribal Population and Prevalence of Hypertension among Adults - Report on Second Repeat Survey. *Technical Report No. 25;* National Institute of Nutrition- Indian Council of Medical Research; NNMB. 2009.

Omron health care. Instruction manual: full body sensor: body composition monitor and scale, *Model HBF,* vol. 510; 2008.

Reddy K. S., Prabhakaran D., Chaturvedi V., et al., Methods for establishing a surveillance system for cardiovascular diseases in Indian industrial populations. *Bulletin of the World Health Organization.* 2006; 84:461-9.

Reddy V. S., Jacob G. P., Ballala K., et al., Study on the prevalence of hypertension among young adults in a coastal district of Karnataka, South India. *International Journal of Healthcare and Biomedical Research*. 2015; b3:32-39.

Rizwan S. A., Kumar R., Singh A. K., et al., Prevalence of hypertension in Indian tribes: a systematic review and meta-analysis of observational studies. *PLoS one*. 2014 May 5; 9(5):e95896.

Sanuade O. A., Boatemaa S., Kushitor M. K. Hypertension prevalence, awareness, treatment and control in Ghanaian population: Evidence from the Ghana demographic and health survey. *PloS one*. 2018 Nov 7; 13(11):e0205985.

Sarkar D., Mondal N., Sen J. Obesity and blood pressure variations among the Bengali Kayastha population of North Bengal, India. *Journal of Life Sciences*. 2009 Jul 1; 1(1):35-43.

Seidell J. C. Waist circumference and waist/hip ratio in relation to all-cause mortality, cancer and sleep apnea. *European journal of clinical nutrition*. 2010 Jan; 64(1):35.

Shakya S., Timilsina M., Timilsina K., et al., Hypertension among young adults in the shopping malls of Kathmandu. *Nepalese Heart Journal.* 2012; 9(1):33-6.

Shanthirani C. S., Pradeepa R., Deepa R., et al., Prevalence and risk factors of hypertension in a selected South Indian population - the Chennai Urban Population Study. *The Journal of the Association of Physicians of India*. 2003 Jan 1; 51:20-7.

Stevens J. P. *Applied multivariate statistics for the social sciences.* Routledge, 2012.

Taing K. Y., Farkouh M. E., Moineddin R., et al., Age and sex-specific associations of anthropometric measures of adiposity with blood pressure and hypertension in India: a cross-sectional study. *BMC cardiovascular disorders*. 2016 Dec; 16(1):247.

World Health Organization 2014. *Global Status Report on Non Communicable Diseases: Attaining the nine global non-communicable diseases targets; a shared responsibility*. 2014.

World Health Organization. *A Global Brief on Hypertension: Silent Killer, Global Public Health Crisis.* Geneva: World Health Organization Press. 2013.

World Health Organization. Burden: Mortality, morbidity and risk factors. *WHO Global Status Report on Non-Communicable Diseases.* WHO. 2010. P. 9-31.

World Health Organization. *Obesity, preventing and managing the global epidemic [Report of a WHO consultation on obesity]*. Geneva: World Health Organization. 1998.

World Health Organization. *Waist circumference and waist-hip ratio: Report of a WHO expert consultation.* Geneva; 2008.

Yusuf S., Rangarajan S., Teo K., et al., Cardiovascular risk and events in 17 low-, middle-, and high-income countries. *New England Journal of Medicine.* 2014 Aug 28; 371(9):818-27.

Zhou Z., Hu D., Chen J. Association between obesity indices and blood pressure or hypertension: which index is the best? *Public health nutrition*. 2009 Aug; 12(8):1061-71.

In: Ethnicity and Syndrome X
Editors: M. Das and K. Bose
ISBN: 978-1-53618-042-8
© 2020 Nova Science Publishers, Inc.

Chapter 11

CARDIO-METABOLIC RISK AMONG THE HIGH ALTITUDE INHABITANTS: A BRIEF REVIEW

***Sovanjan Sarkar*[1] *and Mithun Das*[2,*]**
[1]Department of Anthropology, Vidyasagar University,
Midnapore, West Bengal, India
[2]Department of Anthropology & Tribal Studies,
Sidho-Kanho-Birsha University, Purulia, West Bengal, India

The syndrome X or metabolic syndrome is a cluster of interrelated physiopathological comorbidities identified as a risk factor for cardiovascular disease (CVD) and type 2 diabetes or non-insulin dependent diabetes mellitus (NIDDM) (Wilson et al., 2005). These factors include obesity (especially central adiposity), hyperglycemia, dyslipidemia and hypertension (Grundy et al., 2005). Therefore, this syndrome requires a multiple approach due to its complex and uncertain causes (Grundy et al., 2005; Alberti et al., 2009). The prevalence of syndrome X is increasing all

[*]Corresponding Auhtor's Email: mithundas01@yahoo.com.

over the world, closely related to higher obesity and sedentary lifestyle pattern (Alberti et al., 2009). Thus the syndrome X is a public health problem, which could be reduced by means of healthy lifestyle, policies, and programs (Lucini et al., 2016). Despite the fact that some risk factors for developing syndrome X are widely recognized (e.g., smoking, unhealthy dietary habits, sedentary behavior) (Grundy et al., 2005), insufficient reports about protective factors, such as healthier dietary patterns (Abete et al., 2010), can be found. Concerning modifiable factors, the environment has been suggested to potentially influence the development of metabolic diseases (Friel et al., 2011; Dhurandhar and Keith, 2014; Valdes et al., 2014). Over the past several years prevalence of the syndrome X has also been described in populations with ethnic and cultural differences. Differences in genetic background, diet, levels of physical activity, population age and gender structure, levels of over and undernutrition, and body composition all influence the prevalence of both the syndrome X and its components (Cameron et al., 2004).

It is estimated that over 400 million people worldwide reside in high-altitude areas above 1500 m. High-altitude environment affects the incidence of syndrome X from multiple aspects. First of all, people living in high-altitude areas tend to be leaner when compared with those living in low-altitude areas, and this inverse association is independent of lifestyle, ethnicity and income (Woolcott et al., 2014). Second, as obesity is a well-established risk factor for type 2 diabetes, the less prevalent in obesity can explain the lower prevalence of NIDDM at higher altitudes (Woolcott et al., 2015).Third, there is a positive correlation between altitude and the prevalence of hypertension (Mingji et al., 2015). Fourth, several epidemiological investigations suggest that high altitudes could be associated with dyslipidemia (Hirschler, 2016). Due to the above comprehensive impact on the components of syndrome X, it is difficult to estimate the prevalence of syndrome X at high altitude in theory (Huang et al. 2020).

Living at high altitude has long been studied in relation to human health. It has been suggested that high altitude can affect a range of diseases, either negatively (mainly circulatory or pulmonary disease) (Peacock, 2008;

Mohanna et al., 2006), or positively (diabetes and hypertension) (Baracco et al., 2007). A number of studies in different geographic areas (i.e., USA, Latin America, Asia, and Europe) investigated one or more CVD risk factors among high-altitude residents, but with controversial results. Some of these studies reported that the prevalence of hypertension at high-altitude residents was lower than in low-altitude ones (Wolf et al., 1994; Fiori et al., 2000; Mirrakhimov et al., 1985). Furthermore, cholesterol levels decreased with increasing altitude, whereas high-density lipoprotein cholesterol (HDLc) seemed to be increased (Fioro et al., 2000; Sharma, 1990; Fujimoto et al., 1989; Dominguez et al., 2000; De Mendoza et al., 1979). However, other studies reported opposite results, according to which high-altitude living was associated with elevated blood pressure and increased risk of atherosclerotic disease (Jefferson et al., 2002; Pasini et al., 1999; Temte, 1996). In a study from Peru it was found that the prevalence of syndrome X was higher, even though not significantly, in high-altitude residents compared to those living at low altitude (Baracco et al., 2007). It showed that a considerable proportion of elderly participants have the syndrome X, with those living at high altitudes appearing to have almost double the risk for the syndrome. In a study among the Greek Mediterranean islands, multi-adjusted analysis revealed that elders living at high altitudes islands was associated with higher odds of the syndrome X, irrespective of age, sex, education status, smoking, dietary habits, or physical activity. In addition, elders living at high altitude had higher prevalence of hypercholesterolemia, hypertension, and almost double the burden of obesity than residents in low-altitude (sea level) areas. However, detailed analyses showed that the access to health care is the decisive parameter when studying the prevalence of the syndrome X in the context of altitude of living. The association between living at high altitude and prevalence of the syndrome X was not significant when the annual number of visits to health care centers was included in the analysis. The association remains significant when the mere presence of health care centers, physician offices, or hospitals were taken into account (Tyrovolas et al., 2011). The confounding role of annual number of visits to health care centers on the relationship between altitude and likelihood of syndrome X could imply that it is not the altitude *per se* that contributes to the development of syndrome X, but the lack of opportunity of access to health care for a better control of predisposing factors (blood pressure and lipids levels, weight control, etc). The impact of medical care and control of risk factors on health status seem to be much greater than that of altitude of living. People living in high-altitude areas had a higher prevalence of the syndrome X than those living in low-altitude areas, a fact that can be explained by the under supply of adequate health care services in altitude areas. The latter underlines the need for immediate measures for health promotion among elders living in mountainous and rural areas (Tyrovolas et al., 2011). Whereas, some studies on subjects living at high altitudes have reported lower incidence rates of conditions linked to syndrome X such as obesity (Voss et al., 2013; Woolcott et al., 2014; Diaz-Gutierrez et al., 2016), heart disease (Ezzati et al., 2012; Faeh et al., 2016), hypertension (Norboo et al., 2015) or type 2 diabetes (Woolcott et al., 2014).

Several trials have assessed the role of hypoxia on metabolic and physiologic characteristics (Millet et al., 2016). For instance, body weight was significantly lower in obese subjects exposed to hypobaric hypoxia at geographical altitude (Lippl et al., 2010; Vats et al., 2013). Furthermore, increased basal metabolic rate and leptin levels together with decreased food intake and diastolic blood pressure have been associated with the exposure to higher altitudes (Westerterp-Plantenga et al., 1999; Lippl et al., 2010). These clinical trials suggest that not only normobaric hypoxic exposures, but also hypobaric hypoxia could drive some beneficial effects commonly associated with living at geographical altitude. Some studies have reported beneficial effects of a short-term geographical altitude exposure in subjects with syndrome X (Schobersberger et al., 2003; Greie et al., 2006; Neumayr et al., 2014; Gutwenger et al., 2015). On the other hand, some investigations have reported non-significant changes in obesity or CVD risk factors in obese individuals treated with sham intermittent hypoxia during exercise (Gonzalez- Muniesa et al., 2015b,c; Gatterer et al., 2015) or without exercise (Querido et al., 2012). Likewise, the effects of exercise recovery in hypobaric hypoxia were analyzed with no statistically significant results (Gatterer et al., 2015). Few studies have observed a reduction in body weight of obese subjects treated with physical exercise under normobaric intermittent hypoxia compared to sham hypoxia group (Netzer et al., 2008; Kong et al., 2014). However, higher oxygen availability has been related with beneficial effects in several clinical disorders with an underlying inflammatory cause (Gonzalez-Muniesa et al., 2015a). In a prospective study the association between living at different altitudes and the risk of syndrome X in healthy participants was analyzed in order to evaluate the longitudinal long-term association between altitude of residence and incidence of syndrome X in a cohort of Spanish university graduates (Diaz-Gutierrez et al. 2016). It has been found that living at geographically higher altitude was significantly associated with a decreased risk of developing syndrome X, and this effect followed a linear trend.

The higher concentration of oxygen (O_2) that can be found in the earth corresponds to sea level (21%). At this altitude level the O_2 partial pressure (pO_2) is around 160mm Hg. Every 300m reduces the pO_2 1% (McElroy et al., 2000; West, 2002). It is suggested that living at moderately geographical altitude where the participants are exposed to lower pO_2 pressure, humidity and temperature has a potential preventive effect. The prevalence of obesity has been positively associated with ambient temperature in two different observational studies (Valdes et al., 2014; Yang et al., 2015). A significant reduction in the risk of developing syndrome X associated with living at geographically higher altitudes was found. The outcome was only statistically significant for the syndrome X as a whole but not for each one of its components separately. This lack of significance might be explained by the low incidence of the criteria of syndrome X in this young cohort (1.3% hypertriglyceridemia, 4.0% low HDL-c, 6.7% hypertension, and 2.5% type 2 diabetes). Only central adiposity showed a relatively high incidence in this cohort (27.2%). The reduction in the risk of developing syndrome X living at geographical high altitude followed a similar trend to the main analysis in those subjects with no family history of chronic diseases. It indicates that the genetic background of chronic disease does not interfere with the potential benefits of living at geographical high altitude. Several observational studies have reported lower incidence rates of metabolic diseases in different large cohorts (Ezzati et al., 2012; Voss et al., 2013, 2014; Woolcott et al., 2014; Faeh et al., 2016) living at high altitudes.

Obesity was significantly higher at lower altitude category (<500m) in an US cross-sectional study after controlling for urbanization, temperature, behavioral and demographic factors (males and females had 5.1 and 3.9 times the odds of obesity, respectively, compared to participants over 3000 m) (Voss et al., 2013). A study about the incidence of overweight/obesity at geographical altitude performed in the SUN cohort found a reduction in the risk of developing overweight or obesity (Diaz-Gutierrez et al., 2016). Lately, a quasi-experimental study carried out with military population observed that individuals with frequent migration stationed at high altitude had 41% lower risk of obesity after multiple adjustments (Voss et al., 2014). Another trial, also performed in a US population, observed a lower risk of developing both obesity and type 2 diabetes (OR: 0.77 and 0.88 respectively) at high altitudes (from 1500 to 3000 m) (Woolcott et al., 2014). In addition, two studies found an inverse association between altitude (more than 1500 m) and mortality from ischemic heart disease, while a positive association was established between altitude and mortality from chronic obstructive pulmonary disease (Ezzati et al., 2012). The mortality rate from coronary heart disease was also reduced in men living above 1220m (Faeh et al., 2016). These outcomes are consistent with the results, although they enrolled participants living at considerably higher altitudes than those in the cohort (up to 3500m vs. < 2000 m). Higher hypertension prevalence was associated to highest altitudes (more than 2000m) in highlanders of India (Norboo et al., 2015), which opposed the results concerning hypertension, as the study was carried out with very high altitude dwellers.

With a view to assess the relative roles of environmental (modernization) vis-à-vis genetic factors in the determination of syndrome X and other known risk factors of CVD, we undertook a study (Sarkar et al., 2005; Sarkar et al., 2006) among two tribal groups of India - Toto and Bhutia - who share a common ancestry and live in a similar ecological habitat (rural sub-Himalayan region). A large fraction of one tribe (Bhutia) has adopted a modern life style and lives in an urban area. The *a priori* expectation, if indeed environmental factors are of primary importance, is that the prevalence of dyslipidaemia, diabetes and syndrome X will be low and of similar magnitude among the Toto and rural Bhutia (since these are traditional societies) and higher among the urban Bhutia. If genetic factors are important, then the Toto and rural Bhutia will have prevalence of asimilar magnitude (because of shared ancestry).This study of two tribal populations, believed to have descended from a common ancestral population and resident in the same ecological region (sub-Himalayan region) of India, has been conducted to investigate the possible influence of genetic and environmental factors on parameters of cardiovascular risk (blood pressures, blood lipids, blood glucose and obesity). It is to be noted that even though the two populations share a common genetic ancestry, they have experienced markedly dissimilar socio-demographic histories. Bhutia showed a relatively more adverse cardiovascular risk profile compared to the Toto, as measured by blood pressure, blood lipids and blood glucose. Bhutia had higher mean values in majority of the traits considered, except high density lipoprotein cholesterol (HDLc), irrespective of age groups and gender. Urban Bhutia had generally higher values compared to rural Bhutia, irrespective of gender. The Bhutia -both males and females, and both rural and urban -had a much higher prevalence of syndrome X compared to the Toto. The prevalence of syndrome X was not significantly higher among urban Bhutia compared to their rural counterparts. When Toto and rural Bhutia were compared, the rural Bhutia showed significantly higher values of all variables, except triglycerides (TG) that underlie the definition of syndrome X. Statistically significant differences existed between the Toto and the rural Bhutia in respect of TG, very low density lipoprotein cholesterol (VLDLc) and fasting blood glucose (FBG). While mean TG and VLDLc values in younger as well as older age groups were higher among the Toto as compared with the Bhutia, the reverse was true in case of FBG. This indicates that triglyceridaemia poses a problem among the Toto. On the contrary, among the Bhutia hyperglycaemia was prevalent.Urban Bhutia significantly differed from their rural counterparts in respect of LDLc, VLDLc, TG and FBG. Urban Bhutia had higher mean values compared to rural Bhutia in respect of all these traits in both younger and older age groups, except in FBG. Our study revealed that syndrome X (or its contributing variables) could be a major health problem even in traditional rural ethnic living in different altitudes of the sub-Himalayan regions. It is therefore indicating that this syndrome was not necessarily a result of modernization or urbanization. Further, our study indicated that genetic factors that adversely affect the levels of such variables have long antiquities in Indian ethnic groups. An additional adverse impact of adoption of urban life styles (perhaps primarily mediated through dietary changes) was also apparent on cardiovascular risk factors and syndrome X (Sarkar et al., 2005; Sarkar et al., 2006).

In a small-scale survey of Tibetan immigrants in India, it has been found that the main metabolic abnormalities were obesity and hypertension, while the prevalence of dyslipidaemia and hyperglycaemia was relatively low at high altitude. Finding shows that the prevalence of obesity did not match the prevalence of hyperglycemia at higher altitude. The reasons could be attributed to the cellular response to chronic hypoxia at high altitude may enhance cellular glucose uptake, glycolysis and glycogenesis, but decrease hepatic gluconeogenesis. As a result, it leads to decrease in blood glucose, hemoglobin A1C and increase insulin sensitivity. Moreover, the cold weather and chronic hypoxia at high altitude cause calorie intake increase and energy expenditure decrease, which eventually leads to positive energy gain, and induces overweight and obesity (Lin et al., 2017). Although living in altitude affected the risk of different components of syndrome X, there was no dose–response effect between altitude and the risk of syndrome X due to the opposite effect of altitude on hypertension, obesity and dyslipidaemia as mentioned by Huang et al. (2020). The overall prevalence of syndrome X in high altitude farmers and herdsmen in Tibet was lower compared to other high altitude natives, while its components (hyperglycemia, obesity, and high blood pressure) were higher than in other high altitude communities. Implications of the findings of high prevalence of smoking (among men), obesity, and hypertension and low rates of awareness, treatment, and control of the components of the syndrome X among rural highlanders propels the need for health programs targeting risk factors (Sherpa et al., 2013). In another study among the Tibetan Immigrants living in high altitude areas in Ladakh, India it was found that women have had a higher prevalence of obesity and syndrome X than men. However no relationship was found between diabetes and obesity (Lin et al.,

2017).Among the people living at high altitude in the Peruvian Central Andes it was found that the non HDLc fraction and triglycerides are directly associated to hemoglobin value, and increases in them are in turn associated with higher diastolic blood pressure (Gonzales & Tapia, 2013). Studies show that higher hemoglobin levels, seen in subjects less adapted to altitude, are associated with higher serum total and non-HDL cholesterol and triglyceride levels (Reeves et al., 2004; Wu et al., 2006; Gonzalez, 2011; Gonzalez et al., 2009). This has been shown by controlling confounding variables such as BMI, a marker of anthropometric nutritional status. This would suggest that hypoxemia itself has an impact on lipid profile, particularly on the non-HDL fraction, as opposed to suggestions by other authors that hypercholesterolemia could not be related to altitude hypoxemia (Pajueto et al., 2010; Segura et al., 2006).

High altitude natives are subjected to chronic hypoxia from birth, and this has conditioned a series of adaptive changes, some of which are: metabolic and hormonal changes like lower blood glucose, better and faster glucose uptake in peripheral tissues, higher insulin sensitivity, greater hyperglycemic hormone secretion and caloric expense; and tissue level changes like greater number of capillaries per volume unit in the brain, muscle and myocardium, higher myoglobin and a higher hematocrit (Zubiate, 2001). The Quechua, for instance, settled at high altitude at least 10,000 years ago (Cleeman, 2001), unlike other population groups of different origins. As part of their adaptation they depend on plants and animals to produce meals with a high caloric content, and on the intake of great quantities of carbohydrates (Toselli et al., 2001). Studies done in the past have found that coronary heart disease is less frequent in the high altitude native (Garmendia, 1992); whereas a studydone in Cuzco, Peru (3380 meters above sea level) found a stroke prevalence rate close to that of developed countries, suggesting that CVD is a health care problem in high altitude populations of Peru, and suggested a relationship between stroke and overweight and/or sedentary lifestyle (Jaillard et al., 1995). Studies showing reliable estimates of cardiovascular related morbidity and mortality in sea-level or high-altitude populations are very few and far between. On the other hand, recent studies done on high-altitude populations have demonstrated low prevalence of diabetes mellitus and hypertension (Seclen et al., 1999; Zubiate, 2001). The higher sensitivity to endogenous insulin presented on high altitude natives compared to sea-level habitants should condition a low prevalence of syndrome X since this syndrome has been associated with hyperinsulinemia and insulin resistance, although this has been debated in an ADA statement (Kahn et al., 2005).

CONCLUSION

The geographical elevation may be an important factor linked to metabolic diseases. The high altitude populations seem to have a lower prevalence of CHD and a higher prevalence of stroke than that of low altitude populations. Cardiovascular risk profiles of high altitude populations may depend on altitude, ethnicity, cultural lifestyle practices, and residential setting (urban or rural). Altitude *per se* could be an important additional risk factor because of its association with blood pressure and cardio-metabolic risk. Different ancestry-related physiological responses to the low oxygen environment at higher altitude may affect cardiovascular health consistent with the evidence of different patterns of cardio-metabolic abnormality. Ethnicity and associated lifestyle or cultural practices (such as salt and alcohol intake, smoking habit) and residential settings (mainly differences in physical activity and fruit and vegetable consumption in urban and rural participants), are therefore seems to be important determinants of cardio-metabolic health for high altitude inhabitants. Hence, it requires serious public health attention.

ACKNOWLEDGMENTS

The authors are grateful to Professors Partha Pratim Majumder, Barun Mukhopadhyay, and Chandra Sekhar Chakrabarti for their untiring guidance in every step of the study conducted among Toto and Bhutia populations.

Indian Council of Medical Research (ICMR), New Delhi and Indian Statistical Institute (ISI), Kolkata are acknowledged for financial support to conduct the study among the Totos and Bhutias.

REFERENCES

Abete I, Astrup A, Martinez JA, Thorsdottir I, Zulet M.A. Obesity and the metabolic syndrome: role of different dietary macronutrient distribution patterns and specific nutritional components on weight loss and maintenance. *Nutr Rev.* 2010. 68,214–231.doi:10.1111/j.1753-4887. 2010.00280.x.

Alberti KG., Eckel RH., Grundy SM, Zimmet PZ, Cleeman JI, Donato KA, et al. Harmonizing the metabolic syndrome: a joint interim statement of the International Diabetes Federation Task Force on Epidemiology and Prevention; National Heart, Lung, and Blood Institute; American Heart Association; World Heart Federation; International Atheroscle-rosis Society; and International Association for the Study of Obesity. *Circulation.* 2009; 120, 1640–1645. doi: 10.1161/CIRCULATION AHA.109.192644.

Baracco R, Mohanna S, Seclen S. A comparison of the prevalence of metabolic syndrome and its components in high and low altitude populations in Peru. *Metab Syndr Relat Disord.* 2007; 5(1):55-62.

Cameron A, Shaw J, Zimmet P. The metabolic syndrome: prevalence in worldwide populations. *Endocrinol Metab Clin North Am.* 2004; 33: 351–375.

Cleeman J. Executive summary of the Third Report of the National Cholesterol Education Expert Panel on Detection, Evaluation, and Treatment of High Blood Cholesterol in Adults (ATP III). *JAMA.* 2001; 285: 1–12.

De Mendoza S, Nucete H, Ineichen E, Salazar E, Zerpa A, Glueck CJ. Lipids and lipoproteins in subjects at 1,000 and 3,500 meter altitudes. *Arch Environ Health.* 1979; 34: 308-311.

Dhurandhar EJ, Keith SW. The aetiology of obesity beyond eating more and exercising less. *Best Pract Res Clin Gastroenterol.* 2014; 28: 533–544. doi:10.1016/j.bpg.2014.07.001.

Diaz-Gutierrez J, Martinez-Gonzalez MA, Pons-Izquierdo JJ, Gonzalez-Muniesa P, Martinez JA, Bes-Rastrollo M. Living at higher altitude and incidence of overweight/obesity: prospective analysis of the SUN Cohort. *PLoS ONE.* 2016; 11:e0164483.doi:10.1371/journal.pone.0164483.

Dominguez Coello S, Cabrera De Leon A, Bosa Ojeda F, Perez Mendez LI, Diaz Gonzalez L, Aguirre-Jaime AJ.High density lipoprotein cholesterol increases with living altitude. *Int J Epidemiol.* 2000; 29: 65-70.

Ezzati M, Horwitz ME, Thomas DS, Friedman AB, Roach R, Clark T, et al. Altitude, life expectancy and mortality from ischaemic heart disease, stroke, COPD and cancers: national population-based analysis of US counties. *J Epidemiol Commun Health.* 2012; 66: e17. doi: 10.1136/jech.2010.112938.

Faeh D, Moser A, Panczak R, Bopp M, Roosli M, Spoerri A, et al. Independent at heart: persistent association of altitude with ischaemic heart disease mortality after consideration of climate, topography and built environment. *J Epidemiol Commun Health.* 2016; 70: 798–806. doi: 10.1136/jech-2015-206210.

Fiori G, Faccini F, Pettener D, Rimondi A, Battistini N, Bedgoni G. Relationships between blood pressure, anthropometric characteristic and blood lipid in high and low altitude population from central Asia. *Ann Hum Biol.* 2000; 27: 19-28.

Friel S, Bowen K, Campbell-Lendrum D, Frumkin H, McMichael AJ, and Rasanathan K. Climate change, non-communicable diseases, and development: the relationships and common policy opportunities. *Annu Rev Public Health.* 2011; 32: 133–147. doi: 10.1146/annurev-publhealth-071910-140612.

Fujimoto N, Matsubayashi K, Miyahara T, Murai A, Matsuda M, Shio H, Suzuki H, Kameyama M, SaitoA, Shuping L. The risk factors for ischemic heart disease in Tibetan highlanders. *Jpn Heart J.* 1989. 30:27-34.

Garmendia F. La influencia de la alturasobre la historia natural de las enfermedades [The influence of height on the natural history of diseases]. *Revista Médica Peruana.* 1992; 64:10.

Gatterer H, Haacke S, Burtscher M, Faulhaber M, Melmer A, Ebenbichler C, et al. Normobaric intermittent hypoxia over 8 months does not reduce body weight and metabolic risk factors-a randomized, single-blind, placebo-controlled study in normobaric hypoxia and normobaric sham hypoxia. *Obes. Facts* 2015; 8: 200–209.doi:10.1159/000431157.

Gonzales GF. Hemoglobina y Testosterona: Importanciaen la aclimatación y adaptación a la altura [Hemoglobin and Testosterone: Importance in acclimatization and adaptation to height]. *Rev Peru Med Exp Salud Pública.* 2011; 28: 92-100.

Gonzales GF, Gasco M, Tapia V, Gonzales-Casta˜neda C. High serum testosterone levels are associated with excessive erythrocytosis of chronic mountain sickness in men. *Am J Physiol Endocrinol Metab.* 2009; 296: E1319-E1325.

Gonzales G.F., Tapia V. Association of high altitude-induced hypoxemia to lipid profile and glycemia in men and women living at 4100m in the Peruvian Central Andes. *Endocrinol Nutr.* 2013; 60: 79-86.

Gonzalez-Muniesa P, Garcia-Gerique L, Quintero P, Arriaza S, Lopez-Pascual A, Martinez JA. Effects of hyperoxia on oxygen-related inflammation with a focus on obesity. *Oxid Med Cell Longev.* 2015: 8957827. doi: 10.1155/2016/8957827.

Gonzalez-Muniesa P, Quintero P, De Andres J, Martinez JA. Hypoxia: a consequence of obesity and also a tool to treat excessive weight loss. *Sleep Breath.* 2015; 19: 7–8. doi: 10.1007/s11325-014-0972-2.

Greie S, Humpeler E, Gunga HC, Koralewski E, Klingler A, Mittermayr M, et al. Improvement of metabolic syndrome markers through altitude specific hiking vacations. *J Endocrinol Invest.* 2006; 29: 497–504. doi: 10.1007/BF03344138.

Grundy SM, Cleeman JI, Daniels SR, Donato KA, Eckel RH, Franklin BA, et al. Diagnosis and management of the metabolic syndrome: an

American Heart Association/National Heart, Lung, and Blood Institute scientific statement: executive summary. *Crit Pathw Cardiol.* 2005; 4: 198–203. doi: 10.1097/00132577-200512000-00018.

Gutwenger I, Hofer G, Gutwenger AK, Sandri M, Wiedermann CJ. Pilot study on the effects of a 2-week hiking vacation at moderate versus low altitude on plasma parameters of carbohydrate and lipid metabolism in patients with metabolic syndrome. *BMC Res Notes.* 2015; 8:103. doi: 10.1186/s13104-015-1066-3.

Hirschler V. Cardiometabolic risk factors in native populations living at high altitudes. *Int J Clin Pract.* 2016; 70: 113–118.

Huang X, Hu Y, Du L, et al. Metabolic syndrome in native populations living at high altitude: a cross-sectional survey in Derong, China. *BMJ Open.* 2020; 10:e032840. doi: 10.1136/bmjopen-2019-032840.

Jefferson JA, Escudero E, Hurtado ME, Kelly JP, Swenson ER, Wener MH, Burnier M, Maillard M, Schreiner GF, Schoene RB, Hurtado A, Johnson RJ. Hyperuricemia, hypertension, and proteinuria associated with high-altitude polycythemia. *Am J Kidney Dis.* 2002; 39: 1135-1142.

Jaillard A, Hommel M, Mazetti P. Prevalence of stroke at high altitude (3380m) in Cuzco, a town of Peru: A population-based study. *Stroke.* 1995; 26: 562–568.

Kahn R, Buse J, Ferrannini E, Stern M. The metabolic syndrome: Time for a critical appraisal. Joint Statement from the American Diabetes Association and the European. Association for the Study of Diabetes. *Diabetes Care.* 2005; 28:2 289–2304.

Kong Z, Zang Y, Hu Y. Normobaric hypoxia training causes more weight loss than normoxia training after a 4-week residential camp for obese young adults. *Sleep Breath.* 2014; 18: 591–597. doi: 10.1007/s11325-013-0922-4.

Lin BY, Genden K, Shen W, et al. The prevalence of obesity and metabolic syndrome in Tibetan immigrants living in high altitude areas in Ladakh, India. *Obes Res Clin Pract.* 2017; 12: 365-371.

Lippl FJ, Neubauer S, Schipfer S, Lichter N, Tufman A, Otto B, et al. Hypobaric hypoxia causes body weight reduction in obese subjects. *Obesity (Silver Spring).* 2010. 18; 675–681. doi: 10.1038/oby.2009.509.

Lucini D, Zanuso S, Solaro N, Vigo C, Malacarne M, Pagani M. Reducing the risk of metabolic syndrome at the worksite: preliminary experience with an ecological approach. *Acta Diabetol.* 2016; 53, 63–71. doi: 10.1007/s00592-015-0744-x.

McElroy MK, Gerard A, Powell FL, Prisk GK, Sentse N, Holverda S, et al. Nocturnal O_2 enrichment of room air at high altitude increases day time O_2 saturation without changing control of ventilation. *High Alt Med Biol.* 2000. 1, 197–206. doi: 10.1089/15270290050144190.

Millet GP, Debevec T, Brocherie F, Malatesta D, Girard O. Therapeutic use of exercising in hypoxia: promises and limitations. *Front Physiol.* 2016; 7: 224. doi: 10.3389/fphys.2016.00224.

Mingji C, Onakpoya IJ, Perera R, et al.Relationship between altitude and the prevalence of hypertension in Tibet: a systematic review. *Heart.* 2015; 101: 1054–1060.

Mirrakhimov MM, Rafibekova ZH, Dzhumagulova AS, Meimanaliev TS, Murataliev TM, ShatemirovaKK.Prevalence and clinical peculiarities of essential hypertension in population living at high altitude. *Cor Vasa.* 1985. 27:23-28.

Mohanna S, Baracco R, Seclen S. Lipid profile, waist circumference, and body mass index in a high altitude population. *High Alt Med Biol.* 2006; 7: 245-255.

Netzer,N.C., Chytra,R., and Kupper,T. (2008).Low intense physical exercise in normobaric hypoxia leads to more weight loss in obese people than low intense physical exercise in normobaric hypoxia. *Sleep Breath.* 12, 129–134. doi: 10.1007/s11325-007-0149-3.

Neumayr G, Fries D, Mittermayer M, Humpeler E, Klingler A, Schobersberger W, et al. Effects of hiking at moderate and low altitude on cardiovascular parameters in male patients with metabolic syndrome: Austrian Moderate Altitude Study. *Wilderness Environ. Med.* 2014. 25, 329–334. doi: 10.1016/j.wem.2014.01.003.

Norboo T, Stobdan T, Tsering N, Angchuk N, Tsering P, Ahmed I, et al. Prevalence of hypertension at high altitude: cross- sectional survey in Ladakh, Northern India 2007-2011. *BMJ Open.* 2015; 5: e007026. doi: 10.1136/bmjopen-2014-007026.

Pajuelo Ramirez J, Sánchez-Abanto J, Arba˜nil-Huamán H. Las enfermedadescrónicas no transmisiblesen el Perú y surelación con la altitude [Noncommunicable chronic diseases in Peru and its relation to altitude]. *Rev Soc Per Medic Int.* 2010; 23: 45-53.

Pasini GF, Donato F, Buizza MA, Fantoni C, Gelatti U, Tani M, Grassi V. Prevalence of risk factors for coronary heart disease in a mountain community in northern Italy. *G Ital Cardiol.* 1999. 29:891-897.

Peacock AJ. Medical problems of high altitude. *J R Coll Physicians Edinb.* 2008. 38:126-128.

Querido JS, Sheel AW, Cheema R, Van Eeden S, Mulgrew AT, Ayas, NT. Effects of 10 days of modest intermittent hypoxia on circulating measures of inflammation in healthy humans. *Sleep Breath.* (2012). 16, 657–662.doi: 10.1007/s11325-011-0555-4.

Reeves JT, León-Velarde F. Chronic mountain sickness: recent studies of the relationship between hemoglobin concentration and oxygen transport. *High Alt Med Biol.* 2004; 5: 147-55.

Sarkar S, Das, M, Mukhopadhyay B, Chakraborty CS, Majumder PP. Prevalence of metabolic syndrome in two tribal populations of sub-Himalayan region of India: Ethnic and Rural-Urban differences. *Am J Hum Biol.* 2005; 17: 814-817.

Sarkar S, Das, M, Mukhopadhyay B, Chakraborty CS, Majumder PP. High prevalence of metabolic syndrome & its correlates in two tribal populations of India & the impact of urbanization. *Indian J Med Res.* 2006; 123: 679-686.

Schobersberger W, Schmid P, Lechleitner M, vonDuvillard SP, Hortnagl H, Gunga HC, et al. Austrian Moderate Altitude Study 2000 (AMAS 2000).The effects of moderate altitude (1,700m) on cardiovascular and metabolic variables in patients with metabolic syndrome. *Eur J Appl Physiol.* 2003; 88: 506–514. doi: 10.1007/s00421-002-0736-8.

Seclén S, Leey J, Villena A, Herrera B, Penacho C, Carrasco A, Vargas R. Prevalencia de Diabetes Mellitus, Hipertensión arterial, Hipercolesterolemia y Obesidad Como Factores de Riesgo Coronario y Cerebrovascular en Población Adulta de la Costa, Sierra y Selva del Perú [Prevalence of Diabetes Mellitus, Hypertension,

Hypercholesterolemia and Obesity as Coronary and Cerebrovascular Risk Factors in Adult Population of the Coast, Sierra and Jungle of Peru]. *Acta Medica Peruana.* 1999; 17.

Segura L, Agusti R, Parodi J, Investigadores del studio TORNASOL. Factores de riesgo de las enfermedadescardiovascularesen el Perú (Estudio TORNASOL) [Risk factors for cardiovascular diseases in Peru (TORNASOL Study)]. *Rev Per Cardiol.* 2006; 32: 82-128.

Sharma S. Clinical, biochemical, electrocardiographic and noninvasive hemodynamic assessment of cardiovascular status in natives at high to extreme altitudes (3000m-5500m) of the Himalayan region. *Indian Heart J.* 1990; 42: 375-379.

Sherpa LY, Deji HS, Virasakdi C, Per N, Espen B. Prevalence of metabolic syndrome and common metabolic components in high altitude farmers and herdsmen at 3700 m in Tibet. *High Alt Med Biol.*2013; 14: 37–44.

Temte JL. Elevation of serum cholesterol at high altitude and its relationship to hematocrit. *Wilderness Environ Med.* 1996; 7: 216-224.

Toselli S, Tarazona-Santos E, Pettener D. Body size, composition, and blood pressure of high-altitude Quechua from the Peruvian Central Andes (Huancavelica, 3,680m). *Am J Hum Biol.* 2001; 13: 539–547.

Tyrovolas S, Chalkias C, Morena M, et al. Health care access and prevalence of the Metabolic Syndrome among elders living in high altitude areas of the Mediterrean Islands: The MEDIS Study. *The Review of Diabetic Research.* 2011; 8: 468-476.

Valdes S, Maldonado-Araque C, Garcia-Torres F, Goday A, Bosch-Comas A, Bordiu E, et al. Ambient temperature and prevalence of obesity in the Spanish population: the Diabetes study. *Obesity (Silver Spring)* 2014; 22: 2328–2332. doi: 10.1002/oby.20866.

Vats P, Ray K, Majumadar DA, Joseph DA, Bayen S, et al. Changes in cardiovascular functions, lipid profile, and body composition at high altitude in two different ethnic groups. *High Alt Med Biol.* 2013;14: 45–52. doi: 10.1089/ham.2012.1071.

Voss JD, Masuoka P, Webber BJ, Scher AI, Atkinson RL. Association of elevation, urbanization and ambient temperature with obesity prevalence in the United States. *Int J Obes.* 2013; 37: 1407–1412. doi: 10.1038/ijo.2013.5.

West JB. Commuting to high altitude: value of oxygen enrichment of room air. *High Alt Med Biol.* 2002; 3: 223–235. doi: 10.1089/152702 90260131948.

Wilson PW, D'Agostino RB, Parise H, Sullivan L, Meigs B. Metabolic syndrome as a precursor of cardiovascular disease and type 2 diabetes mellitus. *Circulation.* 2005; 112: 3066–3072. doi: 10.1161/CIRCUL ATIONAHA.105.539528.

Westerterp-Plantenga MS, Westerterp KR, Rubbens M, Verwegen CR, Richelet JP, Gardette B. Appetite at "high altitude" [Operation Everest III (Comex-'97)]: a simulated ascent of Mount Everest. *J Appl Physiol.* 1985. 87, 391–399.

Wolf EE, Selland MA, Mazzeo RS, Reeves JT. Systemic hypertension at 4,300 m is related to sympathoadrenal activity. *J Appl Physiol.*1994. 76:1643-1650.

Woolcott OO, Castillo OA, Gutierrez C, et al. Inverse association between diabetes and altitude: a cross-sectional study in the adult population of the United States. *Obesity.* 2014; 22: 2080–2090.

Woolcott OO, Ader M, Bergman RN. Glucose homeostasis during short-term and prolonged exposure to high altitudes. *Endocr Rev.* 2015; 36: 149–173.

Wu T, Kayser B. High altitude adaptation in Tibetans. *High Alt Med Biol.* 2006; 7: 193-208.

Yang HK, Han K, Cho JH, Yoon KH, Cha BY, Lee SH. Ambient temperature and prevalence of obesity: a Nationwide Population Based Study in Korea. *PLoS ONE.* 2015; 10: e0141724. doi: 10.1371/journal. pone. 0141724.

Zubiate M. SíndromeMetabólico. *Diagnóstico.* 2001; 40: 157–166.

EDITORS' CONTACT INFORMATION

Mithun Das, PhD.,
Associate Professor in Anthropology & Tribal Studies,
Sidho-Kanho-Birsha University, Purulia, West Bengal, India

Kaushik Bose, PhD., DSc.,
Professor, Department of Anthropology,
Vidyasagar University

INDEX

#

21st century, 23, 28, 29

A

access, 48, 84, 86, 122, 130, 142, 183, 197
accounting, 94, 140, 163
acculturation, 32, 36, 37, 38, 39, 40, 41, 42, 44, 45, 135, 150, 176
adaptation, 36, 90, 189, 193, 198
adipokine, 154, 156
adiponectin, 2, 154, 155, 160
adipose, 2, 12, 27, 40, 142, 154, 157, 158, 159, 176
adipose tissue, 2, 27, 40, 142, 154, 157, 158, 159, 176
adiposity, 10, 11, 16, 21, 43, 130, 133, 140, 142, 143, 155, 156, 160, 168, 173, 175, 177, 179, 181, 185
adjustment, 118, 136, 139, 155, 156
adolescents, 2, 8, 18, 22, 28, 30, 33, 34, 41, 43, 76, 77, 78, 79, 80, 81, 82, 83, 85, 89, 90, 176
adulthood, x, 34, 122
adults, 2, 5, 7, 8, 11, 12, 15, 20, 28, 29, 42, 45, 53, 56, 94, 106, 107, 110, 111, 112, 125, 139, 146, 172, 176, 178
affluence, 10, 14, 29, 104
Africa, v, x, 5, 7, 22, 29, 33, 47, 48, 50, 52, 54, 55, 109
African-American, 14, 159, 161
age, xii, 2, 8, 11, 26, 27, 28, 30, 33, 34, 35, 50, 52, 53, 59, 64, 65, 67, 73, 78, 79, 81, 83, 84, 85, 87, 90, 94, 95, 100, 103, 108, 119, 130, 134, 138, 141, 148, 166, 168, 170, 172, 177, 178, 182, 183, 187
American Heart Association, 17, 105, 111, 160, 167, 191, 194
apolipoprotein B, 153
artery, 4, 49, 149, 161
Asia, 5, 7, 16, 35, 40, 46, 59, 77, 115, 122, 125, 127, 146, 147, 150, 183, 192
Asian countries, 4, 139, 143
assessment, 4, 22, 57, 91, 103, 127, 161, 197
assimilation, 33, 34, 44
atherogenic dyslipidemia, 13, 142, 153
atherosclerosis, ix, 18, 53, 157
atherosclerotic, 18, 53, 55, 138, 154, 183

atherosclerotic cardiovascular disease, 18, 154
ATP, 3, 24, 95, 96, 97, 98, 99, 100, 101, 102, 103, 107, 110, 111, 191
awareness, xii, 6, 13, 67, 135, 148, 158, 175, 178, 179, 188

B

Bangladesh, v, x, 57, 58, 60, 62, 63, 64, 67, 68, 69, 70, 71, 72, 73, 127
behaviors, 18, 89, 135, 136
benefits, 6, 13, 157
biomarkers, xii, 155, 158
birth weight, x, 11, 38, 59, 132
blood, xi, 1, 12, 27, 28, 29, 51, 52, 55, 56, 78, 85, 107, 117, 118, 126, 134, 137, 139, 142, 145, 147, 150, 153, 163, 167, 168, 170, 172, 173, 174, 175, 176, 178, 179, 180, 183, 187, 188, 189, 190, 192, 197
blood pressure, xi, 1, 2, 11, 29, 35, 40, 51, 55, 56, 78, 85, 117, 118, 125, 126, 134, 137, 139, 142, 145, 147, 150, 153, 163, 167, 168, 169, 170, 171, 172, 173, 175, 176, 178, 179, 180, 183, 184, 187, 188, 190, 192, 197
body composition, x, 10, 21, 125, 133, 159, 164, 168, 172, 173, 175, 177, 179, 182, 197
body fat, 6, 118, 119, 126, 142, 154, 156, 164, 167, 169, 171, 173, 177
body image, 18, 22
body mass index, 3, 19, 20, 21, 28, 46, 62, 73, 115, 125, 127, 155, 159, 164, 168, 169, 171, 178, 195
body mass index (BMI), 3, 4, 10, 19, 20, 21, 28, 46, 62, 73, 76, 78, 80, 84, 96, 115, 118, 119, 120, 121, 125, 126, 127, 135, 155, 156, 159, 161, 164, 168, 169, 171, 172, 173, 176, 177, 178, 189, 195
body size, 14, 16, 22
body weight, 27, 76, 126, 184, 193, 194
Brazil, 5, 7, 8, 13, 20, 21, 49, 76, 122, 175

C

CAD, 4, 49, 94
calorie, 6, 143, 188
cancer, 26, 27, 94, 115, 179
carbohydrate(s), 6, 141, 189, 194
cardiovascular disease(s), vi, xi, 1, 18, 20, 21, 26, 27, 35, 45, 54, 94, 95, 108, 114, 127, 129, 131, 137, 140, 143, 144, 146, 154, 160, 176, 177, 179, 181, 197, 198
cardiovascular risk, 5, 11, 14, 17, 45, 49, 55, 126, 132, 137, 138, 145, 147, 149, 150, 154, 161, 187
Census, 72, 116, 125
central obesity, 17, 26, 28, 49, 55, 114, 118, 125, 126, 142, 143, 174
challenges, 28, 55, 71, 144
Chicago, 126, 168, 178
childhood, x, 5, 11, 21, 33, 42, 43, 46, 54, 59, 89, 122, 125
children, 5, 6, 8, 11, 12, 14, 15, 16, 22, 28, 30, 33, 34, 41, 43, 46, 48, 51, 58, 60, 62, 69, 72, 75, 76, 77, 78, 79, 80, 81, 82, 83, 84, 85, 86, 89, 90, 91, 108, 137
China, 4, 7, 9, 12, 19, 20, 29, 35, 76, 87, 112, 194
chi-square test, 58, 64, 67
cholesterol, ix, xi, 1, 6, 22, 27, 49, 53, 56, 96, 107, 111, 125, 138, 142, 154, 183, 187, 189, 191, 192, 197
chronic diseases, xii, 8, 9, 12, 18, 23, 26, 28, 115, 138, 144, 155, 167, 185, 196
chronic hypoxia, 188, 189
cigarette smoking, 4, 51, 54
cities, 7, 13, 14, 48, 90, 104
clustering, 14, 19, 27, 49, 94, 114
colon, ix, 27, 161

community/communities, 5, 12, 14, 15, 22, 41, 44, 52, 53, 55, 57, 67, 68, 69, 71, 104, 107, 109, 110, 111, 117, 130, 144, 145, 147, 164, 175, 188, 196
complications, ix, 17, 54, 105, 130
composition, 133, 155, 173, 197
consensus, 27, 106, 107, 138
consumption, ix, 6, 7, 39, 58, 122, 125, 135, 137, 138, 190
cooperation, 105, 124, 145
coronary artery disease, 4, 49, 94, 149, 161
coronary heart disease, 4, 16, 22, 27, 51, 52, 55, 56, 109, 141, 186, 189, 196
correlation, 4, 39, 118, 139, 157
C-reactive protein, x, 23, 49, 154, 159, 160, 161
cross sectional study, 72, 111, 147
cross-sectional study, 16, 42, 102, 104, 107, 112, 115, 147, 150, 155, 166, 180, 186, 198
CRP, 154, 155, 157
CVD, xii, 1, 4, 6, 8, 9, 12, 15, 94, 115, 118, 137, 140, 181, 183, 184, 186, 189
cytokines, 2, 154, 157

D

data collection, 63, 124, 174
DBP, 78, 82, 83, 168, 169
deaths, 9, 26, 59, 114, 163
deficiency/deficiencies, 12, 59, 68
demographic, 10, 56, 61, 62, 64, 65, 66, 67, 68, 71, 72, 73, 103, 110, 119, 131, 133, 136, 177, 179, 186, 187
demographic factors, 62, 66, 67, 186
demographic transition, 10
deposition, 10, 90, 142, 173, 174
detection, xii, 56, 176
developed countries, 5, 9, 12, 14, 131, 135, 139, 189
developing countries, 5, 6, 7, 8, 9, 10, 11, 12, 13, 14, 15, 17, 18, 19, 21, 49, 55, 58, 73, 93, 113, 114, 131, 137, 143, 149, 164
diabetes, vi, ix, xi, xii, 1, 4, 9, 10, 16, 19, 21, 22, 23, 26, 27, 28, 30, 34, 35, 36, 37, 38, 39, 40, 42, 43, 44, 45, 46, 49, 52, 55 94, 95, 96, 105, 106, 107, 108, 110, 111, 114, 115, 127, 129, 131, 132, 134, 135, 138, 139, 141, 142, 144, 145, 146, 147, 148, 149, 150, 155, 158, 159, 160, 161, 176, 177, 181, 182, 183, 185, 186, 188, 190, 191, 194, 196, 197, 198
diabetes mellitus, 29, 34, 43, 49, 52, 105, 142, 147, 149, 190
diagnostic criteria, 95, 96, 97, 98, 99, 101, 103
diastolic blood pressure, 29, 50, 168, 169, 184, 189
diastolic blood pressures, 50
diet, 13, 18, 20, 23, 36, 43, 44, 58, 89, 114, 124, 144, 178, 182
dietary habits, 5, 105, 182, 183
dietary patterns, 7, 54, 182
diseases, ix, x, xii, 5, 6, 8, 9, 10, 11, 12, 15, 16, 19, 21, 25, 26, 27, 29, 32, 33, 37, 39, 43, 55, 104, 108, 113, 114, 122, 127, 131, 137, 143, 144, 149, 155, 173, 180, 182, 185, 190, 192, 193
disorder, 45, 115, 142
distribution, 154, 156, 173, 191
dyslipidemia, 10, 13, 26, 27, 49, 93, 96, 114, 142, 153, 181, 182

E

economic status, 11, 13, 51, 54, 63, 64, 65, 66, 117
economy, 6, 13, 14, 48, 55
education, 34, 62, 64, 67, 70, 131, 176, 183
energy, 7, 21, 34, 36, 38, 39, 68, 143, 159, 188

environment(s), 12, 15, 34, 36, 37, 38, 39, 43, 56, 77, 86, 91, 130, 131, 132, 133, 134, 135, 136, 140, 141, 143, 144, 182, 190, 192
environmental factors, 3, 12, 15, 50, 88, 91, 186
epidemic, 21, 38, 44, 55, 105, 111, 127, 139, 180
epidemiologic, 10, 25, 39, 44, 55, 156
epidemiologic transition, 10, 25, 39, 44
epidemiology, 107, 109, 144, 149
ethnic groups, x, xi, xii, 2, 6, 10, 43, 64, 114, 127, 142, 155, 156, 188, 197
ethnicity/ethnicities, v, x, xi, xii, 1, 2, 3, 15, 16, 27, 39, 42, 43, 114, 121, 123, 154, 155, 158, 164, 166, 182, 190
Europe, 29, 33, 34, 35, 36, 45, 140, 183
evidence, 5, 10, 11, 42, 71, 148, 155, 190
exposure, 54, 143, 184, 198

F

factor analysis, 176, 177, 178
family history, x, 4, 52, 155, 159, 185
famine, 6, 11, 26, 36
fasting, 2, 22, 27, 138, 141, 155, 187
fasting blood glucose, 27, 187
fat, 6, 7, 10, 23, 34, 36, 38, 76, 90, 115, 141, 142, 147, 154, 156, 158, 164, 167, 169, 171, 173, 174
food, ix, 7, 8, 10, 11, 12, 13, 15, 17, 18, 20, 34, 39, 41, 43, 58, 83, 84, 125, 136, 139, 141, 184
Ford, 27, 41, 93, 107

G

gender, 2, 3, 17, 22, 27, 41, 85, 130, 136, 138, 146, 154, 158, 159, 176, 177, 182, 187
genetic factors, 11, 35, 36, 50, 89, 143, 186
genetic predisposition, 134, 137, 144
genotype, 10, 43, 143
glucose, ix, 2, 12, 21, 27, 28, 38, 141, 142, 143, 153, 157, 187, 188, 189
growth, 6, 14, 28, 38, 58, 73, 76, 77, 81, 88, 91, 133
guidelines, 18, 100, 101, 102, 104, 118, 126, 167, 178

H

habitat(s), 13, 30, 131, 132, 133, 186
Hawaii, 35, 147, 149
hazards, 37, 134, 135
health, ix, x, xi, xii, 5, 8, 12, 15, 22, 23, 26, 27, 31, 32, 33, 37, 39, 40, 41, 42, 43, 44, 45, 48, 54, 58, 60, 68, 69, 70, 71, 72, 73, 93, 109, 112, 113, 114, 115, 118, 122, 124, 130, 131, 134, 135, 136, 137, 139, 144, 146, 147, 148, 149, 150, 155, 160, 163, 174, 179, 180, 182, 183, 187, 188, 189, 190
health care, 54, 70, 94, 136, 179, 183, 189, 197
health condition, 130, 132, 134, 144, 174
health education, 12, 15, 70, 144
health status, 114, 130, 131, 134, 136, 164, 174, 184
heart attack, ix, 26, 94, 163
heart disease, 4, 16, 22, 27, 51, 52, 55, 56, 109, 141, 184, 186, 189, 193, 196
height, 28, 59, 62, 73, 76, 77, 78, 79, 83, 90, 117, 118, 119, 124, 125, 126, 164, 166, 167, 168, 169, 171, 176, 178, 193
high blood pressure, 2, 29, 35, 125, 135, 142, 168, 170, 171, 172, 176, 188
high density lipoprotein, xi, 1, 142, 154, 187, 192
high density lipoprotein cholesterol, xi, 1, 142, 154, 187, 192

high-altitude, 182, 183, 189, 194, 197
Hispanics, xi, 2, 45, 156
history, x, 4, 28, 30, 44, 52, 53, 143, 155, 159, 185, 193
homeostasis, 22, 157, 198
host, 32, 33, 35, 37, 131, 132, 143, 157
host population, 32, 35, 131, 132
human, x, 6, 11, 21, 43, 48, 73, 75, 88, 129, 133, 138, 144, 182
humidity, 185
hyperglycaemia, 187, 188
hyperglycemia, xi, 1, 11, 28, 114, 142, 181, 188
hyperinsulinemia, 11, 24, 49, 190
hyper-insulinemia, 114
hypertension, vi, ix, x, 11, 13, 26, 27, 29, 30, 34, 35, 38, 40, 41, 42, 45, 49, 50, 51, 52, 53, 54, 55, 56, 93, 96, 113, 114, 115, 118, 119, 121, 122, 123, 124, 125, 126, 127, 129, 131, 132, 134, 136, 139, 141, 143, 144, 145, 146, 147, 148, 150, 151, 163, 164, 168, 170, 171, 172, 173, 174, 175, 176, 177, 178, 179, 180, 181, 182, 183, 185, 188, 190, 194, 195, 196, 198
hypertriglyceridemia, 11, 26, 52, 185
hypobaric, 184, 194
hypothesis, 11, 18, 32, 36, 38, 155
hypoxemia, 189, 193
hypoxia, 184, 188, 189, 193, 194, 195, 196

I

ideal, 54, 118, 134
identification, 10, 30, 62, 104
immigrants, 33, 34, 35, 40, 41, 42, 43, 45, 139, 140, 149, 188, 194
immigration, 31, 41, 46
in situ urbanization, 14
in utero, 11, 37, 143
incidence, 35, 41, 51, 52, 54, 94, 138, 160, 177, 182, 184, 185, 192
income, 7, 9, 13, 26, 29, 30, 35, 37, 38, 39, 47, 48, 59, 68, 90, 108, 131, 134, 135, 149, 180, 182
India, vi, x, 1, 4, 5, 7, 8, 9, 12, 14, 17, 18, 19, 21, 23, 29, 33, 35, 40, 42, 60, 93, 94, 96, 99, 100, 103, 104, 105, 106, 107, 108, 109, 110, 111, 112, 113, 115, 125, 129, 136, 140, 143, 145, 146, 147, 153, 155, 163, 164, 165, 170, 171, 172, 173, 174, 175, 176, 177, 178, 179, 180, 181, 186, 188, 194, 195, 196, 199
Indians, vi, x, 4, 14, 16, 17, 21, 23, 24, 39, 49, 51, 52, 53, 55, 56, 107, 110, 114, 129, 131, 134, 137, 142, 155, 176
individuals, 2, 4, 6, 11, 28, 62, 94, 118, 120, 130, 132, 135, 136, 139, 140, 141, 142, 144, 154, 184, 186
inequality, 48, 83
infection, 56, 113, 156
inflammation, 16, 142, 154, 156, 157, 158, 159, 160, 161, 193, 196
inflammatory markers, 49, 154
insulin, ix, 11, 13, 16, 19, 20, 22, 23, 28, 38, 49, 52, 55, 138, 140, 141, 142, 147, 155, 156, 157, 158, 159, 160, 188, 189
insulin resistance, 11, 13, 16, 19, 23, 28, 49, 52, 55, 138, 140, 141, 142, 155, 157, 158, 159, 160, 190
insulin sensitivity, 188, 189
interleukin-6, 154
intervention, xii, 5, 12, 57, 70, 104, 141, 144
Iran, 4, 8, 16, 109
Islam, v, 41, 72, 73, 140, 141, 147
issues, 58, 60, 130, 133, 136, 144, 164

K

kidney, 29, 94, 163

L

later life, 34, 37, 39, 140, 143
Latin America, 5, 7, 183
lead, 4, 28, 38, 42, 54, 77, 115, 163
leptin, 154, 158, 160, 177, 184
life expectancy, 10, 29, 114, 192
lifestyle, 5, 6, 10, 11, 12, 13, 15, 21, 34, 37, 40, 44, 54, 103, 110, 112, 114, 115, 127, 130, 133, 134, 136, 139, 140, 141, 142, 143, 144, 149, 154, 156, 163, 173, 182, 190
lifestyle changes, 6, 21, 127, 154
lifestyle transitions, 10
lipid abnormalities, 54
lipids, 89, 142, 184, 187, 191
lipoprotein abnormalities, 153
liver, ix, 94, 142, 156, 157, 177
living conditions, 37, 77, 85, 130
low density lipoprotein cholesterol, 153

M

magnitude, 27, 103, 135, 137, 143, 154, 186
majority, 15, 31, 34, 48, 117, 144, 187
malnutrition, 20, 21, 38, 58, 59, 69, 72, 73
management, xii, 17, 125, 158, 193
marriage, 62, 64, 65, 66, 67
mass, 6, 54, 85, 126, 154, 176, 177
measurement, 117, 127, 167, 178
measurements, 21, 78, 117, 166, 168
medical, 25, 29, 30, 48, 72, 95, 112, 176, 178, 184
medicine, ix, 90, 177, 178
Mediterranean, 29, 33, 35, 42, 183
mellitus, xi, 1, 26, 29, 34, 39, 43, 45, 49, 52, 105, 142, 147, 149, 158, 181, 190, 198
mental health, 32, 45, 148
meta-analysis, 103, 148, 175, 179
Metabolic, vi, 17, 44, 45, 49, 93, 95, 96, 97, 104, 106, 107, 108, 109, 110, 111, 112, 114, 126, 129, 142, 145, 159, 160, 161, 177, 181, 194, 197, 198
metabolic disorder(s), ix, x, 131, 137, 138, 139, 142, 144, 159
metabolic syndrome, vi, ix, x, xi, 1, 17, 18, 19, 20, 22, 23, 24, 26, 39, 43, 44, 45, 49, 93, 94, 95, 96, 97, 100, 101, 102, 103, 104, 105, 106, 107, 108, 109, 110, 111, 112, 114, 118, 125, 126, 129, 134, 137, 138, 142, 143, 145, 149, 151, 154, 159, 160, 161, 176, 177, 181, 191, 193, 194, 195, 196, 197, 198
metabolism, 10, 38, 71, 142, 157, 161
meter, 28, 167, 191
Middle East, 7, 8, 10, 33, 35, 149
migrant population, 13, 32, 136, 138
migrants, 5, 31, 32, 33, 34, 35, 36, 37, 38, 40, 42, 43, 45, 46, 129, 131, 133, 135, 137, 138, 140, 142, 144, 147, 148, 149, 150
migration, v, vi, x, 5, 12, 14, 15, 25, 26, 30, 31, 32, 33, 36, 37, 38, 39, 40, 42, 43, 48, 87, 104, 129, 131, 133, 134, 136, 137, 138, 140, 143, 144, 145, 146, 147, 148, 150, 151, 186
minorities, 43, 45, 149
modernization, 5, 36, 37, 38, 131, 135, 163, 186
Mongolia, x, 75, 77, 85, 86, 87, 88, 90
morbidity, 12, 15, 25, 32, 34, 43, 51, 57, 59, 94, 108, 109, 115, 141, 143, 180, 189
mortality, 8, 9, 10, 12, 15, 19, 25, 34, 35, 43, 44, 51, 52, 57, 59, 94, 108, 109, 115, 125, 130, 141, 143, 179, 180, 186, 189, 192
mortality rate, 35, 52, 186
Moscow, 75, 86, 87, 88, 89, 90

N

National Cholesterol Education Program Adult Treatment Panel-III, 95
National Family and Health Survey, 115
neolithic transition, 25
Netherlands, 35, 40, 41, 42
Nigeria, 50, 76, 106
non-communicable diseases, 25, 26, 32, 33, 37, 104, 114, 127, 131, 137, 144, 180, 192
non-insulin dependent diabetes mellitus, 142, 181
normobaric, 184, 193, 194, 195
North America, xi, 107, 176
nutrition, 5, 6, 10, 12, 13, 15, 17, 18, 20, 21, 23, 37, 39, 43, 44, 57, 58, 60, 62, 66, 67, 68, 70, 71, 73, 91, 113, 125, 137, 141, 143, 177, 178, 179, 180
nutrition transition, 5, 6, 10, 12, 13, 15, 18, 20, 21, 44, 125, 137
nutritional status, x, 58, 59, 60, 62, 63, 64, 66, 67, 68, 69, 70, 71, 127, 144, 189

O

O2 partial pressure, 185
obesity, vi, ix, xi, 1, 2, 3, 5, 6, 8, 9, 10, 11, 12, 13, 14, 15, 16, 17, 18, 19, 20, 21, 22, 23, 26, 27, 28, 30, 33, 34, 35, 36, 37, 38, 39, 40, 41, 42, 43, 44, 45, 46, 49, 51, 52, 53, 55, 89, 93, 96, 105, 113, 114, 115, 118, 122, 124, 125, 126, 127, 130, 132, 135, 139, 140, 141, 142, 143, 144, 146, 147, 148, 149, 150, 154, 155, 156, 158, 159, 160, 161, 164, 167, 173, 174, 177, 179, 180, 181, 182, 183, 184, 185, 187, 188, 191, 192, 193, 194, 197, 198
opportunities, 31, 34, 192
overnutrition, 12, 15, 20
overweight, x, 6, 8, 18, 28, 33, 34, 36, 40, 41, 42, 43, 45, 46, 115, 118, 119, 121, 122, 123, 124, 125, 130, 164, 186, 188, 189, 192
oxygen, 185, 190, 193, 196, 198

P

Pacific, xi, 16, 29, 35, 40, 42, 127
parents, 14, 67, 84
participants, 69, 100, 117, 124, 135, 166, 167, 171, 174, 183, 185, 190
PCA, 168, 170, 172
Peru, 76, 138, 148, 149, 183, 189, 191, 193, 194, 196, 197
phenotype(s), 6, 10, 11, 18, 21, 38, 131, 139, 144, 147, 154
physical activity, 4, 5, 6, 8, 10, 12, 13, 15, 16, 19, 20, 22, 23, 34, 36, 37, 42, 76, 84, 89, 137, 141, 146, 149, 182, 183, 190
physical exercise, 13, 85, 184, 195
physical fitness, 85, 86, 88
physical inactivity, ix, 7, 8, 17, 19, 20, 34, 35, 39, 135, 139, 142, 143, 149
pilot study, 22, 109, 147
plasma glucose, 12, 153
PM, 39, 55, 161
Poland, x, 91, 147, 150
policy, 20, 54, 145, 146, 149, 174, 192
polycystic ovarian syndrome, 94
population, xii, 2, 3, 5, 6, 8, 11, 13, 14, 16, 18, 19, 20, 21, 22, 24, 27, 29, 31, 35, 47, 48, 50, 51, 52, 53, 54, 56, 60, 61, 64, 66, 67, 68, 72, 73, 77, 88, 90, 93, 94, 100, 104, 106, 108, 109, 110, 111, 112, 114, 115, 116, 118, 119, 125, 126, 130, 131, 133, 135,136, 137, 139, 140, 142, 143, 144, 146, 147, 150, 151, 155, 164, 165, 168, 171, 172, 174, 176, 177, 178, 179, 182, 186, 187, 189, 192, 194, 195, 197, 198

population group, 52, 114, 137, 164, 174, 189
poverty, 30, 31, 34, 38, 48, 60, 140, 143
pregnancy, 19, 23, 38, 59
premature death, 29, 59, 163
preschool, 9, 16, 59, 62
preschool children, 9, 16, 59
prevalence rate, 100, 122, 189
prevention, xi, xii, 2, 21, 23, 53, 54, 127, 147, 149, 158, 176
programming, 12, 21, 37
proinflammatory state, 153, 154, 157, 158
project, 34, 86, 175
public health, ix, xi, xii, 28, 59, 93, 112, 124, 137, 144, 160, 180, 182, 190
public services, 48

Q

questionnaire, 63, 69, 117, 166

R

researchers, x, 61, 70, 77, 84, 95, 130, 132, 135, 136, 139, 141, 142, 174
resistance, 16, 19, 20, 49, 51, 52, 56, 141, 142
resources, 31, 83, 132
response, 12, 50, 140, 154, 157, 166, 188
risk(s), ix, x, xi, xii, 1, 2, 3, 8, 10, 11, 12, 13, 14, 15, 16, 17, 18, 19, 20, 21, 22, 26, 27, 29, 30, 32, 33, 34, 35, 38, 40, 41, 42, 45, 49, 52, 53, 54, 55, 58, 73, 89, 94, 96, 107, 109, 110, 112, 114, 115, 118, 121, 122, 125, 126, 132, 135, 136, 137, 138, 140, 141, 142, 143, 144, 145, 146, 147, 149, 151, 153, 154, 155, 157, 161, 163, 164, 172, 173, 174, 176, 177, 178, 179, 180, 181, 182, 183, 184, 185, 186, 188, 190, 192, 193, 194, 195, 196
risk factors, xi, 1, 2, 3, 10, 11, 13, 14, 16, 18, 19, 20, 26, 27, 30, 34, 40, 41, 45, 49, 52, 53, 54, 55, 89, 96, 107, 109, 110, 112, 114, 115, 122, 125, 126, 136, 137, 138, 140, 144, 146, 147, 149, 151, 153, 154, 157, 163, 173, 176, 178, 179, 180, 182, 183, 184, 186, 188, 192, 193, 194, 196
risk profile, 4, 114, 133, 187, 190
rural areas, 8, 13, 14, 58, 60, 76, 83, 132, 133, 135, 138, 140, 143, 184
rural population, 75, 77, 85, 111, 112, 140, 176
Russia, 35, 75, 76, 88, 90

S

school, 9, 15, 48, 67, 84, 90
sea level, 183, 185, 189
sedentary behavior, 89, 163, 182
sedentary jobs, 13
sedentary lifestyle, 6, 140, 143, 144, 182, 189
sensitivity, 157, 188, 189
serum, 49, 50, 53, 141, 142, 153, 155, 157, 189, 193, 197
services, 36, 48, 70, 130, 184
SES, 10, 11, 13
sex, x, 2, 15, 28, 52, 53, 73, 78, 116, 130, 138, 155, 166, 170, 179, 183
showing, 8, 156, 189
skinfolds, 117, 166, 167, 168, 169, 171
smoking, 4, 13, 51, 52, 53, 54, 122, 135, 137, 182, 183, 188, 190
society, 37, 38, 60, 68, 114
socioeconomic status, 34, 36, 37, 39, 41, 46
sodium, 50, 55, 135
South Africa, v, x, 22, 47, 48, 50, 51, 52, 54, 55, 56, 109

South Asia, xi, 2, 7, 10, 19, 29, 52, 55, 59, 95, 106, 114, 126, 137, 144, 146, 148, 149, 150
Spring, 18, 158, 194, 197
standard deviation, 59, 80, 118, 168
starvation, 28, 31, 36
state, 27, 41, 52, 55, 77, 100, 103, 115, 116, 153, 154, 156, 157, 158, 178
states, 76, 156, 165
statistics, 109, 110, 118, 120, 168
storage, 8, 36, 38
stress, 6, 10, 12, 15, 32, 36, 39, 85, 86, 136, 143, 158
stroke, ix, 26, 109, 110, 115, 141, 163, 189, 190, 192, 194
structure, 54, 84, 182
style(s), x, 26, 32, 36, 38, 39, 84, 186, 188
subcutaneous adipose tissue, 155, 176
sub-Saharan Africa, 7, 10, 48, 51
susceptibility, 2, 3, 17, 134, 140, 143
symptoms, ix, 26, 27, 28, 30, 37
syndrome, ix, x, xi, xii, 1, 2, 3, 5, 6, 9, 10, 11, 12, 15, 16, 17, 18, 19, 20, 22, 23, 24, 26, 27, 29, 30, 34, 36, 37, 38, 39, 43, 44, 45, 49, 93, 94, 95, 96, 100, 101, 102, 103, 104, 105, 106, 107, 108, 109, 110, 111, 112, 114, 125, 126, 134, 137, 138, 142, 143,145, 149, 151, 154, 155, 156, 157, 158, 159, 160, 161, 176, 181, 182, 183, 184, 185, 186, 188, 190, 191, 193, 194, 195, 196, 197, 198
syndrome X, v, vi, ix, x, xi, xii, 1, 2, 3, 5, 6, 9, 10, 11, 12, 15, 25, 26, 27, 29, 30, 34, 36, 37, 38, 47, 49, 51, 93, 114, 153, 154, 155, 156, 157, 158, 159, 181, 182, 183, 184, 185, 186, 188, 190
systolic blood pressure(s), 11, 29, 40, 50, 135, 139, 168, 169

T

Task Force, 105, 127, 191
temperature, 185, 197, 198
thrifty genotype, 10, 21, 43
thrifty phenotype, 11, 18, 21, 38
Tibet, 188, 195, 197
tissue, 2, 142, 154, 156, 157, 158, 189
training, 15, 84, 86, 194
transformation(s), 20, 83, 132, 133
transport, 9, 50, 196
treatment, xii, 51, 54, 56, 68, 135, 148, 158, 160, 176, 179, 188
Tribal Rajshahi district, 58
triglyceridaemia, 52, 187
triglycerides, ix, xi, 1, 3, 49, 142, 187, 189
tuberculosis, 55, 72, 146
tumor necrosis factor-α, 154
Turkey, 8, 16, 33, 35, 41, 151
type 2 diabetes, xi, 1, 21, 22, 26, 36, 39, 42, 43, 45, 46, 150, 158, 181, 182, 184, 185, 198
type 2 diabetes mellitus, xi, 1, 26, 39, 45, 94, 158, 198

U

undernutrition, vi, 5, 11, 12, 15, 20, 39, 59, 71, 113, 115, 119, 122, 125, 126, 127, 177, 182
United Kingdom, 35, 43, 140
United States (USA), 2, 22, 31, 33, 34, 35, 39, 40, 46, 52, 55, 73, 95, 139, 141, 168, 183, 198
urban, 5, 7, 8, 11, 12, 13, 14, 15, 18, 19, 21, 22, 23, 31, 48, 50, 51, 54, 55, 56, 69, 75, 76, 77, 78, 79, 80, 81, 82, 83, 84, 85, 86, 87, 89, 90, 91, 95, 104, 105, 106, 107, 109, 110, 111, 130, 131, 133, 134, 136,

137, 139, 140, 141, 143, 144, 145, 146, 147, 148, 149, 151, 175, 177, 186, 190
urban areas, 7, 31, 132, 134, 136, 138
urban population, 54, 90, 105, 107, 133, 138, 141
urbanization, 5, 10, 13, 14, 21, 36, 77, 86, 103, 104, 111, 114, 131, 133, 135, 137, 140, 143, 144, 150, 186, 188, 196, 197

V

variables, 63, 69, 119, 130, 139, 168, 170, 172, 173, 176, 187, 196
variations, 81, 127, 144, 155, 156, 179
vascular diseases, 134, 135, 137, 139, 141, 142, 157
very low density lipoprotein cholesterol, 187
visceral adipose tissue, 154

W

waist circumference, 27, 28, 119, 120, 156, 164, 166, 167, 168, 169, 171, 175, 177, 178, 179, 180, 195
waist girth, 2, 3
waist hip ratio, 164, 168, 169, 171
Washington, 18, 22, 73
weight loss, 28, 191, 193, 194, 195
weight status, 28, 37, 155
workers, 73, 148, 175
World Bank, 48, 55, 72, 73
World Health Organisation (WHO), ix, 4, 9, 13, 17, 23, 24, 26, 27, 28, 29, 46, 49, 54, 58, 59, 72, 73, 95, 96, 97, 98, 99, 100, 101, 103, 105, 107, 114, 118, 125, 127, 163, 173, 179, 180
worldwide, x, xii, 9, 28, 29, 30, 31, 39, 44, 46, 106, 107, 115, 140, 142, 163, 173, 182, 191

Y

young adults, 21, 30, 44, 173, 179, 194